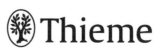

Drug-Induced Sleep Endoscopy

Diagnostic and Therapeutic Applications

Nico de Vries, MD, PhD
Professor of Otorhinolaryngology
Department of Otorhinolaryngology, Head and Neck Surgery
OLVG West Hospital;
Department of Oral Kinesiology
Academic Centre for Dentistry Amsterdam
MOVE Research Institute Amsterdam
University of Amsterdam and VU University Amsterdam
Amsterdam, The Netherlands;
Department of Otorhinolaryngology, Head and Neck Surgery
Antwerp University Hospital (UZA)
Antwerp, Belgium

Ottavio Piccin, MD
Professor of Otorhinolaryngology
Department of Otolaryngology, Head and Neck Surgery
Sant'Orsola-Malpighi University Hospital
Bologna, Italy

Olivier M. Vanderveken, MD, PhD
Chair and Professor of Otorhinolaryngology
Translational Neurosciences
University of Antwerp
Antwerp, Belgium;
Department of Otolaryngology, Head and Neck Surgery
Antwerp University Hospital (UZA)
Edegem, Belgium

Claudio Vicini, MD
Chief of Head and Neck Department
AUSL Romagna;
Head of ENT Units
Forli and Faenza;
Associate Professor of Otolaryngology
University of Ferrara and Bologna
Bologna, Italy

81 illustrations

Thieme
Stuttgart • New York • Delhi • Rio de Janeiro

Library of Congress Cataloging-in-Publication Data

Names: Vries, N. de (Nico), editor. | Piccin, Ottavio, editor. |
    Vanderveken, Olivier M., editor. | Vicini, Claudio, editor.
Title: Drug-induced sleep endoscopy : diagnostic therapy and thera-
    peutic applications / [edited by] Nico de Vries, Ottavio Piccin,
    Olivier M. Vanderveken, Claudio Vicini.
Description: New York, NY : Thieme, [2020] | Includes bibliographical
    references and index. | Summary: "Obstructive sleep apnea is the
    most prevalent sleep-related breathing disorder, impacting an esti-
    mated 1.36 billion people worldwide. In the past, OSA was almost
    exclusively treated with Continuous Positive Airway Pressure
    (CPAP), however, dynamic assessment of upper airway obstruction
    with Drug-Induced Sleep Endoscopy (DISE) has been instrumental
    in developing efficacious alternatives. Drug-Induced Sleep Endos-
    copy: Diagnostic and Therapeutic Applications by Nico de Vries,
    Ottavio Piccin, Olivier Vanderveken, and Claudio Vicini is the first
    textbook on DISE written by world-renowned sleep medicine
    pioneers"– Provided by publisher.
Identifiers: LCCN 2020040346 (print) | LCCN 2020040347 (ebook) |
    ISBN 9783132403468 (hardback) | ISBN 9783132403666 (ebook)
Subjects: MESH: Sleep Apnea, Obstructive–therapy |
    Endoscopy–methods
Classification: LCC RC547 (print) | LCC RC547 (ebook) | NLM WF 145 |
    DDC 616.8/49807545–dc23
LC record available at https://lccn.loc.gov/2020040346
LC ebook record available at https://lccn.loc.gov/2020040347

© 2021. Thieme. All rights reserved.

Georg Thieme Verlag KG
Rüdigerstrasse 14, 70469 Stuttgart, Germany
+49 [0]711 8931 421, customerservice@thieme.de

Thieme Publishers New York
333 Seventh Avenue, New York, NY 10001 USA
+1 800 782 3488, customerservice@thieme.com

Thieme Publishers Delhi
A-12, Second Floor, Sector-2, Noida-201301
Uttar Pradesh, India
+91 120 45 566 00, customerservice@thieme.in

Thieme Publishers Rio, Thieme Publicações Ltda.
Edifício Rodolpho de Paoli, 25º andar
Av. Nilo Peçanha, 50 - Sala 2508
Rio de Janeiro 20020-906 Brasil
+55 21 3172 2297 / +55 21 3172 1896

Cover design: Thieme Publishing Group
Typesetting by TNQ Technologies, India

Printed in Germany by CPI Books

ISBN 978-3-13-240346-8

Also available as an e-book:
eISBN 978-3-13-240366-6

Important note: Medicine is an ever-changing science undergoing continual development. Research and clinical experience are continually expanding our knowledge, in particular our knowledge of proper treatment and drug therapy. Insofar as this book mentions any dosage or application, readers may rest assured that the authors, editors, and publishers have made every effort to ensure that such references are in accordance with **the state of knowledge at the time of production of the book**.

Nevertheless, this does not involve, imply, or express any guarantee or responsibility on the part of the publishers in respect to any dosage instructions and forms of applications stated in the book. **Every user is requested to examine carefully** the manufacturers' leaflets accompanying each drug and to check, if necessary in consultation with a physician or specialist, whether the dosage schedules mentioned therein or the contraindications stated by the manufacturers differ from the statements made in the present book. Such examination is particularly important with drugs that are either rarely used or have been newly released on the market. Every dosage schedule or every form of application used is entirely at the user's own risk and responsibility. The authors and publishers request every user to report to the publishers any discrepancies or inaccuracies noticed. If errors in this work are found after publication, errata will be posted at www.thieme.com on the product description page.

Some of the product names, patents, and registered designs referred to in this book are in fact registered trademarks or proprietary names even though specific reference to this fact is not always made in the text. Therefore, the appearance of a name without designation as proprietary is not to be construed as a representation by the publisher that it is in the public domain.

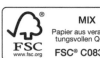

Contents

Videos

Edited by Pien Bosschieter

Representative examples of the most common forms of obstruction during drug-induced sleep endoscopy (DISE), according to velum, oropharynx, tongue base, and epiglottis (VOTE) classification, are shown in this video library.

Examples include the different levels, severity and configuration of obstruction and the effects of chin lift and head rotation.

Velum

Video 1: Complete anteroposterior obstruction at velum level and the effect of jaw thrust and head and trunk rotation.
Video 2: Partial concentric obstruction at velum level.
Video 3: Complete concentric obstruction at velum level and the effect of jaw thrust.

Oropharynx

Video 4: Complete lateral obstruction at oropharynx level caused by enlarged tonsils.
Video 5: Complete lateral obstruction at oropharynx level without enlarged tonsils.

Tongue Base and Epiglottis

Video 6: Complete anteroposterior obstruction at tongue base and epiglottis level and the effect of jaw thrust and head and trunk rotation.
Video 7: Partial anteroposterior obstruction on tongue base and epiglottis.
Video 8: Complete anteroposterior obstruction caused by floppy epiglottis and the effect of head and trunk rotation and jaw thrust.
Video 9: Complete concentric collapse. (Video provided courtesy of Prof. Clemens Heiser.)
Video 10: Trans oral DISE to evaluate the tongue-palate potential interaction, which is difficult to detect while looking at the airway from behind.

Preface

Obstructive sleep apnea (OSA) is the most prevalent sleep-related breathing disorder. Diagnostic workup originally consisted of medical history taking and routine clinical examination followed by a sleep study, which was during the time that OSA was almost exclusively treated with continous positive airway pressure (CPAP). Treatment of OSA is, however, gradually but consistently moving away from CPAP only, and we are presently living in an era of treatment diversification. Many different forms of treatment are now available. Treatment with CPAP has reached a certain plateau, but important innovations have taken place in other therapies, while still other treatments are in development. Next to CPAP, conservative treatment modalities include oral appliance therapy and positional therapy in positional OSA and weight loss—either conservative or by means of bariatric surgery—while surgical approaches consist of all variations of ENT upper airway surgery, maxillofacial surgery, and upper airway stimulation. These alternative treatments ask for additional diagnostic workup. In particular, in upper airway surgery and upper airway stimulation, detailed endoscopic assessment of the collapsible segment of the upper airway, during sleep, is mandatory. Since it is difficult, time-consuming, and labour-intensive to perform endoscopy of the upper airway during natural sleep, the procedure is usually performed during artifically induced sleep. Various names have been proposed for the procedure, but it is presently known as drug induced sleep endoscopy (DISE). Upper airway surgery and upper airway stimulation, as a rule, should not be performed without DISE first. More controversial is the use of DISE in case of oral appliance therapy, positional therapy, or when combination therapy is considered.

Drug Induced Sleep Endoscopy is the first monograph on this exciting and relatively new topic. After a short introduction, DISE in historical perpective is discussed by Prof. Bhik Kotecha and coworkers. Prof Kotecha, at The Royal National Throat, Nose and Ear Hospital, London, works in the institute where DISE was first developed. Subsequently, applicability, indications, contraindications, informed consent, organization and logistics, patient preparation, drugs for DISE, predictive value of DISE and different manouvres during the procedure, complications, DISE and position dependency, significance of complete concentric collapse, collapse of the epiglottis, mistakes in DISE, role of DISE in therapeutic decision-making, DISE and oral appliances, DISE and upper airway stimulation, pediatric DISE, DISE and craniofacial syndromes, and advanced techniques are all discussed. Finally, a comprehensive video library with common and rare DISE findings is included.

We are confident that the book will serve as a guide for beginners in DISE and also hope that experienced endoscopists will find it to be of value. We welcome all valuable comments and suggestions. All authors either have a clinical (DISE) and/or scientific research background. They have spent a great amount of effort on this book, which has made this publication possible. Our deepest gratitude to all our friends who aided us in this great endeavor!

Nico de Vries, MD, PhD
Ottavio Piccin, MD
Olivier M. Vanderveken, MD, PhD
Claudio Vicini, MD

Contributors

Vikas Agrawal, MBBS, MS,DORL, FCPS
Consultant ENT and Sleep Apnea Surgeon;
Director
Speciality ENT Hospital
Mumbai, India

Riccardo Albertini, MD
Resident
Department of Otolaryngology Head and Neck Surgery
Sant'Orsola-Malpighi University Hospital
Bologna, Italy

Annemieke M.E.H. Beelen, MD
Department of Otorhinolaryngology Head and Neck
Surgery
Onze Lieve Vrouwe Gasthuis (OLVG)
Amsterdam, The Netherlands

Palma Benedek, MD, PhD
Associate Professor
Consultant on Pediatric ENT and Sleep Surgery
Chief of the Pediatric Sleep Laboratory
Heim Pal National Pediatric Institute
Budapest, Hungary

Linda Benoist, MD
Department of Otorhinolaryngology Head and Neck
Surgery
University of Rotterdam
Rotterdam, The Netherlands

Pien Bosschieter, MD
Department of Otorhinolaryngology Head and Neck
Surgery
Onze Lieve Vrouwe Gasthuis (OLVG)
Amsterdam, The Netherlands

Luca Burgio, MD
ENT Physician
Department of Otorhinolaryngology, Head and Neck
Surgery
Maurizio Bufalini Hospital
Cesena, Italy

Marc Blumen, MD
Department of Otolaryngology, Head and Neck Surgery
Foch Hospital
Suresnes, France

An Boudewyns, MD
Faculty of Medicine and Health Sciences
University of Antwerp
Department of ENT Head and Neck Surgery
Antwerp University Hospital
Antwerp, Belgium

Giuseppe Caccamo, MD
Resident
Department of Otolaryngology Head and Neck Surgery
Sant'Orsola-Malpighi University Hospital
Bologna, Italy

Giovanni Cammaroto, MD
Head and Neck Department
ENT and Oral Surgery Unit
G.B. Morgagni – L. Pierantoni Hospital
Forlì, Italy

A. Simon Carney, BSc (Hons), MBChB, FRCS, FRACS, DM
Professor
Department of Otolaryngology Head and Neck Surgery
College of Medicine and Public Health
Flinders University
Adelaide, South Australia, Australia

Peter Catcheside, BSc (Hons), PhD
Professor
Adelaide Institute for Sleep Health
College of Medicine and Public Health
Flinders University
Adelaide, South Australia, Australia

Eleonora Cioccoloni, MD
Consultant
Department of Otolaryngology Head and Neck Surgery
Sant'Orsola-Malpighi University Hospital
Bologna, Italy

R.M. Corso, MD
Operating Room Medical Director
Department of Surgery
Anesthesia and Intensive Care Section
"GB Morgagni-L. Pierantoni" Hospital
Forlì, Italy

Paolo Cozzolino, MD
Resident
Department of Otolaryngology Head and Neck Surgery
Sant'Orsola-Malpighi University Hospital
Bologna, Italy

Nico de Vries, MD, PhD
Professor of Otorhinolaryngology
Department of Otorhinolaryngology Head and Neck
Surgery
Onze Lieve Vrouwe Gasthuis (OLVG);
Department of Oral Kinesiology
Academic Centre for Dentistry Amsterdam
MOVE Research Institute Amsterdam
University of Amsterdam and VU University Amsterdam
Amsterdam, The Netherlands;
Department of Otorhinolaryngology Head and Neck
Surgery
Antwerp University Hospital (UZA)
Antwerp, Belgium

Ida Di Giacinto, MD
Anesthesiologist
Polyvalent Intensive Care and Transplantation Unit
Department of Organ Failure and Transplantation
Sant'Orsola-Malpighi University Hospital;
Alma Mater Studiorum
University of Bologna
Bologna, Italy

M. Boyd Gillespie, MD, MSc
Professor & Chair
Department of Otolaryngology- Head & Neck Surgery
University of Tennessee Health Science Center
Memphis, Tennessee, USA

Riccardo Gobbi, MD
Head and Neck Department
ENT & Oral Surgery Unit
G.B. Morgagni - L. Pierantoni Hospital
Forlì, Italy

Evert Hamans, MD
ENT Surgeon
Ziekenhuis Netwerk Antwerpen
Antwerpen, Belgium

Clemens Heiser, MD
Associate Professor
Department of Otorhinolaryngology
Head and Neck Surgery
Munich Technical University
Munich, Germany

Bhik Kotecha, MBBCh, M Phil., FRCS, DLO
Consultant Otolaryngologist
Royal National Throat, Nose and Ear Hospital;
Hon. Clinical Professor
Barts and The London School of Medicine
London, United Kingdom

Ioannis Koutsourelakis, MD, PhD
Surgeon
ENT Department
Mediterraneo Hospital
Athens, Greece

P. Vijaya Krishnan, MBBS, DNB, DLO, MNAMS
Consultant ENT Surgeon;
Head
Department of Snoring and Sleep Disorders
Madras ENT Research Foundation
Chennai, India

Ivor Kwame, MBBS, BSc, MRCS, DOHNS
Otolaryngology Specialist Registrar Surgeon
Sleep Division
Royal National Throat, Nose, and Ear Hospital
University College London Hospitals
London, United Kingdom

Marina Carrasco Llatas, MD
Department of Ear, Nose, and Throat
Dr. Peset University Hospital
Valencia, Spain

Nadia Mansouri, MD
Department of Oral and Maxillo-Facial Surgery
University of Marrakech Medical School
Marrakesh, Morocco

Andrea Marzetti, MD
Chief of ENT Department Head and Neck Area
Frosinone–Alatri Hospital Group
ASL Frosinone
Frosinone, Italy

Joachim T. Maurer, MD
Sleep Disorders Centre
Department of Otorhinolaryngology
Head and Neck Surgery
University Hospital Mannheim
Mannheim, Germany

Filippo Montevecchi, MD
Consultant
Head and Neck Department
ENT & Oral Surgery Unit
G.B. Morgagni - L. Pierantoni Hospital
Forlì, Italy

Paolo G. Morselli, MD
Professor of Plastic and Reconstructive Surgery
Sant'Orsola-Malpighi University Hospital
Alma Mater Studiorum University of Bologna
Bologna, Italy

Adrian A. Ong, MD
Resident Physician
Department of Otolaryngology
University at Buffalo
The State University of New York
Buffalo, New York, USA

Francesco M. Passali, MD, PhD
Professor
Dept. of Clinical Sciences and Translational Medicine
University of Rome Tor Vergata
Rome, Italy

Irene Pelligra, MD
Depatment of Otolaryngology, Head, and Neck Surgery
Sant'Orsola-Malpighi University Hospital
Bologna, Italy

Eli Van de Perck, MD
Faculty of Medicine and Health Sciences
University of Antwerp, Belgium;
Department of ENT Head and Neck Surgery
Antwerp University Hospital UZA
Antwerp, Belgium

Ottavio Piccin, MD
Professor of Otorhinolaryngology
Department of Otolaryngology, Head and Neck Surgery
Sant'Orsola-Malpighi University Hospital
Bologna, Italy

Valentina Pinto, MD
Plastic and Reconstructive Surgeon
Sant'Orsola-Malpighi University Hospital
Alma Mater Studiorum University of Bologna
Bologna, Italy

Madeline J.L. Ravesloot, MD
Department of Otorhinolaryngology Head and Neck Surgery
Onze Lieve Vrouwe Gasthuis (OLVG)
Amsterdam, The Netherlands

Rossella Sgarzani, MD
Consultant, Plastic and Reconstructive Surgeon
Department of Emergency, Burn Center
Bufalini Hospital
AUSL Romagna
Cesena, Italy

Srinivas Kishore S., MBBS, MS
Head
Department of ENT and Sleep Apnea Surgery
Star Hospital
Hyderabad, India

Massimiliano Sorbello, MD
Anesthesiologist
Anesthesia and Intensive Care
AOU Policlinico Vittorio Emanuele
Catania, Italy

Giovanni Sorrenti, MD
Consultant
Department of Otolaryngology Head and Neck Surgery
Sant'Orsola-Malpighi University Hospital
Bologna, Italy

Olivier M. Vanderveken, MD, PhD
Chair and Professor of Otorhinolaryngology
Translational Neurosciences
University of Antwerp
Antwerp, Belgium;
Department of Otolaryngology, Head and Neck Surgery
Antwerp University Hospital (UZA)
Edegem, Belgium

Claudio Vicini, MD
Chief of Head and Neck Department
AUSL Romagna;
Head
ENT Units, Forli and Faenza;
Associate Professor of Otolaryngology
University of Ferrara and Bologna
Bologna, Italy

Patty E. Vonk, MD
Department of Otorhinolaryngology Head and Neck Surgery
Onze Lieve Vrouwe Gasthuis (OLVG)
Amsterdam, The Netherlands

Anneclaire V.M.T. Vroegop, MD
Faculty of Medicine and Health Sciences
University of Antwerp, Belgium
Department of ENT, Head and Neck Surgery
Antwerp University Hospital (UZA)
Edegem, Belgium

Alex Wall, BSc (Hons) DPS
Medical Device Research Institute
College of Science and Engineering
Flinders University
Tonsley, Australia

1 Introduction

Nico de Vries, Ottavio Piccin, Claudio Vicini, and Olivier M. Vanderveken

Abstract

The two cornerstones of obstructive sleep apnea (OSA) workup are sleep study and drug-induced sleep endoscopy (DISE); the latter comes into play in case alternatives to continuous positive airway pressure (CPAP) therapy are considered. This book provides all information on drug-induced sleep endoscopy that is presently available. Some of the world's key opinion leaders in this field, accumulating a vast experience of tens of thousands of DISE procedures, have collaborated in this project.

Keywords: obstructive sleep apnea, history, drug-induced sleep endoscopy

1.1 Obstructive Sleep Apnea

Obstructive sleep apnea (OSA) is a unique disease in the sense that it is both very commonplace and serious.

Incidence in adults was earlier reported to be 2 to 4% of the adult population but recent research, particularly in Switzerland, has shown that it is actually much higher—up to 49% of the male adult population has an apnea hypopnea index above 5.

OSA complaints include loud snoring, excessive daytime sleepiness, tiredness, concentration loss, impaired intellectual performance, among others. Basically, everything that one can imagine as a consequence of repetitive insufficient good sleep can happen.

OSA consequences are, particularly in advanced disease, increased cardiovascular risk, high blood pressure, weight gain, and higher risk of getting involved in accidents.

While as much as 80% of patients with OSA are undiagnosed, awareness is on the rise.

In case of suspicion of OSA, one starts with meticulous medical history taking. Thereafter, an OSA specific physical examination follows. Subsequently, a form of sleep study is scheduled. This is usually a polysomnography or polygraphy in a sleep laboratory or at home. Although in the past this was often regarded as sufficient information to start treatment with continuous positive airway pressure (CPAP), presently therapies other than CPAP are gaining ground as well. Not surprisingly, in this era of personalized medicine, treatment diversification and shared decision-making, the one-size-fits-all, exclusive concept of CPAP therapy is gradually being abandoned.

Current alternative treatments include oral device treatment, positional therapy in case of positional OSA, weight loss in case of overweight, all forms of upper airway surgery, either at the same time or staged, upper airway stimulation and treatment combinations.

In case surgery is considered, drug-induced sleep endoscopy (DISE) is pivotal and often performed after the sleep study has confirmed the diagnosis of OSA. DISE aims at mimicking the normal situation during sleep as closely as possible. While it is well understood that natural sleep and drug-induced sleep are not the same, there is no other method to assess the severity, level(s), and configuration of obstruction of the upper airway that rivals DISE as a viable alternative. DISE as a selection for surgery however remains somewhat controversial, since DISE opponents argue that the evidence that the results of sleep surgery after DISE are better than surgery without DISE is lacking. It is, in fact, even more controversial if DISE should be performed in case oral device therapy, positional therapy, or combination treatment is considered.

This book aims at providing state-of-the-art information on all aspects of DISE. The book starts with background information and historical perspectives, and continues with indications and contraindications. Many different systems have been described and proposed. Which system(s) are presently considered the most useful and which one is mostly used?

Preparation for DISE and informed consent are highlighted. Periprocedural care as well as equipment and documentation is discussed. Some centers perform hundreds of DISEs per year. In case of high-volume of DISEs, good organization, training, and logistics are crucial. Patient preparation and positioning are important. The choice of medication and drug administration and other anesthesiologic aspects deserve proper attention. Should DISE be performed always in case surgery is considered, or only on indication, and if so, which indications are there? How do DISE findings translate into therapeutic surgical and nonsurgical treatment planning? Is DISE safe? What setting is needed? What are the specific indications and contraindications, which personnel is needed, should it be performed in the OR, or can it be performed in a dedicated endosuite outside the OR complex? Is it necessary that the endoscopist and surgeon are the same? Which medication and in which dosage is recommended?

During the procedure itself, passive maneuvers such as chin lift, jaw trust, mouth closure, and titration bite can be performed. Should all these maneuvers always be performed as a matter of routine? Should DISE be performed only in case upper airway surgery or upper airway stimulation are considered or also in cases in which oral device treatment is considered? What is known about the positive and negative predictive value of a maneuver such as jaw thrust? Should DISE be performed in case positional therapy is considered? While previously it was advised to perform DISE in supine position because the obstruction is in that particular position at its most, it can be argued that it is better to perform DISE in lateral position, in case positional therapy is offered either as monotherapy or combined with another treatment modality, or in both supine and lateral position. What is the predictive value of rotation of the head or both head and trunk during DISE? Rotation of the head is only easier and quicker, but is it the same as rotation of both head and trunk? Is it necessary to assess both left and right lateral position, or is the outcome the same? What is the predictive value of a combination of jaw trust and rotation of the head or both head and trunk in case combined positional therapy and oral device treatment are considered?

Work in progress includes the development of a prediction model for such maneuvers, as a selection tool for oral device therapy and positional therapy. What is the predictive value of a combination of jaw trust and rotation of the head or both head and trunk in case combined positional therapy and oral device treatment are considered?

When DISE is performed *lege artis*, and certain requirements are fulfilled, complications are fortunately extremely rare.

Outcomes of large DISE series are described. Intuitively, no obstruction is better than partial obstruction: partial is better than total, anteroposterior and lateral obstruction are better than concentric, and unilevel is better than multilevel. How do all such findings lead to rational treatment advices? For example, is the advice for surgery of a partial and total collapse of the tongue the same or different? Does multilevel obstruction always implicate multilevel treatment or multilevel surgery, and at the same time or staged? In which situation(s) do DISE findings lead to the advice of not performing upper airway surgery?

Usually, but not always, medical history, results of the sleep study and DISE are inline, for example, a history of mild complaints, and mild-to-moderate OSA in the sleep study, correlates with mild obstruction during DISE (one level of obstruction instead of multilevel, no partial obstruction instead of total obstruction, AP–collapse vs. concentric). On the other hand, a history of severe complaints, moderate-to-severe OSA in the sleep study, usually correlates with convincing collapse patterns as multilevel or even obstruction on all levels, total and concentric. However, sometimes there seems to be a mismatch between medical history, sleep study, and DISE findings. One should be aware of this and, if needed, not hesitate to repeat the particular study (either the sleep study or DISE) that does not seem to make sense.

The significance of special findings such as complete concentric collapse of the palate and epiglottic collapse are highlighted. Complete concentric collapse of the palate is "bad news" for standard palatal surgery, as it is regarded as an absolute contraindication for upper airway stimulation, and results of oral device therapy are less favorable as well. Epiglottis collapse occurs in some 8%, and was long regarded as an important justification to perform DISE anyhow, since the only way to discover it is DISE. Recent research shows that epiglottis collapse almost exclusively occurs during DISE in supine position. The consequences are obvious and important.

An exciting recent development is hypoglossal nerve stimulation. The role of DISE before and after hypoglossal nerve stimulation (in case of unexplained failure of the therapy) is critically appraised. In such a situation, DISE often reveals that the effect of upper airway stimulation on the base of tongue collapse is good, but there is no palatal coupling with residual palatal collapse as a consequence. Additional palatal surgery can be indicated in such a case. Higher and lower power settings and different settings—such as monopolar versus bipolar—can be tested as well and might have important clinical consequences.

DISE can prove to be of value in CPAP titration and in case of unexplained CPAP failure. The role of DISE in craniofacial diseases is discussed as well.

A critical discussion of DISE in children, both from an European perspective as well as a US point of view, follows. What is the role of DISE in OSA among children? What is the difference in the role, findings and therapeutic options of DISE in kids and adults? Are the classification systems for kids and children identical?

The book ends with advanced techniques and future perspectives.

There is no better way to understand DISE than by means of studying DISE videos. An extensive DISE video library is therefore available, including not only examples of the most common findings but also rare conditions and examples of difficult cases with important clinical consequences, for example, is the obstruction during DISE anteroposterior or concentric? Is the patient a suitable candidate for upper airway stimulation?

In sum, the two cornerstones of OSA workup are sleep study and DISE. This book provides all information on DISE that is presently available. We have gathered some of the world's key opinion leaders in the field of DISE, accumulating a vast experience of tens of thousands of DISE procedures in the past decades, and grateful for their effort in collaborating for this important endeavor.

We trust this monograph will serve as a reference guide on when, why and how to perform DISE, how to interpret findings, and how such findings translate into treatment advices, with the belief that this will ultimately lead to better outcomes for our patients.

2 Historical Perspective

Bhik Kotecha and Ivor Kwame

Abstract

In this chapter, we have detailed the evolution of drug-induced sleep endoscopy (DISE) over the last 4 decades. We have discussed its emergence as a way of gaining insight into the anatomic patterns of obstruction associated with sleep-disordered breathing (SDB), and outlined many of the controversies surrounding its genuine representation of natural sleep. We have also highlighted the changes in the use of varied anesthetic agents and monitoring to provide and maintain optimal levels of sedation. Finally, we have outlined the emergence of different grading systems in an attempt to consistently document findings, and touched on the role technology has had in enabling real-time involvement of more members of the operating team.

The developments in the way DISE is conducted, interpreted, and documented have ultimately built on the foundations of using the findings during DISE to better guide appropriate operative and nonoperative treatments in patients with SDB.

Keywords: obstructive sleep apnea, drug-induced sleep endoscopy, history

2.1 Introduction

Drug-induced sleep endoscopy (DISE) allows detailed assessment of the upper airway during pharmacologically simulated sleep. It is a useful investigation in patients with sleep disordered breathing (SDB), including obstructive sleep apnea (OSA) prior to tailored and targeted management.

In this chapter, we will recount the general evolution of sleep endoscopy from its earlier derivatives to its more recognizable current format.

2.2 The Original Concept

2.2.1 Early Work

Whilst DISE is now fairly commonplace, the concept of sleep endoscopy only began to appear in the literature in the late 1970's with the original focus being on endoscopic assessment during natural sleep. In 1978, Borowiecki et al wrote an article outlining a study where 10 patients with confirmed hypersomnia sleep apnea (HAS) had a fiber optic bronchoscope inserted through one topically anesthetized nasal airway and secured in place to view just above the soft palate.[1] The patients were then encouraged to sleep in their natural sleeping position with recordings made of their overnight sleep during which the position of the endoscope was adjusted periodically to assess different aspects of the pharynx and the larynx. Rojewski et al built on this early work with their 1984 publication featuring simultaneous full polysomnography with videoendoscopic recordings of the pharynx, again during natural sleep.[2]

Whilst the work reported by Borowiecki and Rojewski furthered our intrigue and understanding of upper airway dynamics during SDB, they did recognize the limitation that a significant duration of time was necessary to conduct each study in order to evaluate the full night data for meaningful findings. Also, queries continued about whether sleep in a laboratory environment with a foreign body within the nasal airway continues to represent the patient's own natural physiological sleep. This controversy about how closely any endoscopic assessment of sleep truly represents natural physiological sleep continues until today. What is clear is that these studies provided us more insight into the patient's natural sleep behavior, particularly obstructive anatomical events.

2.2.2 The Origins of DISE

The concept of DISE, as we know it, began to emerge in the early 1990's with Croft and Pringle's 1991 publication. Their article featured the use of sedation in SDB patients with simultaneous endoscopic assessment of the upper airway to observe sites of obstruction. Their groundbreaking early work demonstrated the concept that sedation could be a shorter surrogate for physiological sleep, albeit not an identical replication.[3,4,5] A further seven articles followed citing analogous techniques, mostly featuring midazolam as the sedative of choice until the 2000. Thereafter, a plethora of articles emerged describing differences in the anesthetic mix, clinical observations during study, and meaningful grading of the results.[6,7] In the following segments, we will further explore each of these in turn.

2.2.3 History of DISE–Controversies

Two of the greatest controversies of DISE are the validity of its representation of physiological sleep and how consistently observers interpret the same physiological findings. Furthermore, questions have arisen as to which drugs would be ideal in conducting DISE and at what depth of sedation the analysis should take place in order to accurately reflect what happens in natural sleep.

Representation

Over the years, many papers have published studies to help address the issue of how closely sedation mirrors physiological sleep. It is widely accepted that sedation does not feature the rapid eye movement (REM) aspect of natural sleep; however, sedation does induce phases of alertness that mirror components of the sleep cycle. Many cite this parallel as a useful surrogate for sleep, albeit an imperfect reproduction.[6,7,8,9,10] However, other challenges about representation remain, including whether a snapshot of sleep is itself valid, whether sleeping position matters, and what depth of sedation is optimal. We will explore each of these in turn.

It is common to change body positions throughout natural sleep; however, we know from polysomnography that most patients with snoring consistently do so whilst on the backs, albeit not exclusively. For this reason, the accepted practice of DISE has long been for patients to be assessed whilst in a supine position.[7,11,12,13,14] The 2014 European position paper on DISE has further recommended assessment be conducted in the sleeping position most associated with snoring in that patient if objective or patient-reported information indicate that it is not the usual supine position.[6]

We have already discussed that extended whole night physiological studies assessing patterns of upper airway movements were first conducted in the 1970's.[1,2] Whilst these provided useful insight, the volumes of data that then required analysis for each patient made the practice difficult to extrapolate into common clinical practice. It is also argued that whilst such studies may be reflective of natural sleep, they are an imperfect model, as they require the subject to sleep in an unfamiliar environment with a foreign body within their nasal cavity,[11] both of which may affect the patient's sleep. It has also been demonstrated that SDB patients can produce comparable apnea–hypopnea index (AHI) scores with DISE as in their natural sleep.[11]

Polysomnography studies have also demonstrated that physiological sleep typically features a rapid eye movement (REM) stage, suppressed during sedation,[10,11] alongside four recognizable stages, each with distinctive electroencephalogram (EEG) changes. Studies have shown that recognizable NREM1, NREM2, and NREM3 EEG patterns demonstrated in sedation are analogous to those observed in natural states.[10,12] Not all phases of sleep feature obstruction with snoring throughout, even in very symptomatic patients;[11,12,13,14] therefore, anything less than a full and complete sleep cycle would have to be considered a sample, in much the same way as sampling is done in statistical models. However, given the accepted restrictions in time, DISE does possess the benefit that it can bring SDB patients to a timely depth of sedation such that they are able to snore during the period of assessment.[10,11,12,13,14,15] Extended DISE studies have been considered; however, concerns persist that anesthetic risks may increase with significant increases in the duration of assessment.[16] It is interesting that not all SDB patients with reported snoring are able to reproduce snoring during DISE.[13] We will discuss depth of sedation along with the anesthetic agents later in the chapter.

Anesthesia

Recommendations about optimal anesthetic combinations in DISE have been detailed in previous publications[7,10] and are not repeated in this chapter. However, such studies surmise that a level of sedation that renders the patient unaware of their surroundings but not completely unarousable is preferable, as such states produce AHI and EEG patterns most analogous to the patients' natural sleep patterns. Changes in the profiles of anesthetic agents and their delivery systems and monitoring over time have led to greater confidence in achieving desirable sedation levels.

Midazolam, a gamma–aminobutyric acid A (GABA-A) agonist benzodiazepine, featured heavily in initial DISE studies and continues to play a role in the sedation process. Of late, the use of the nonopioid GABA-A agonist Propofol (2–6-diisopropylphenol) has become increasingly popular in DISE with or without the synergistic use of agents such as midazolam or dexmedetomidine, an alpha 2-adrenergic agonist. The choice between which of them is largely based on patient factors and the anesthetist's preference with factors considered including the drugs' tendency to induce apnea or labile blood pressure readings as well as their amnesic and/or analgesic properties.

Beyond the changing trends of anesthetic agents, the underlying principles of anesthesia have also witnessed changes. Early work typically featured giving small boluses of anesthetic with careful physiological (blood-pressure, heart rate, etc.) assessment of responses to determine appropriate sedation levels. However target-controlled infusion (TCI) has become more consistently used and was recommended in the 2014 European position paper.[6] TCI enables the selection of a targeted blood concentration of anesthetic agent, with the drug delivery system producing a corresponding rate of delivery. The concentration target can be adjusted through the procedure to achieve the desired level of sedation.

Another aid to encourage appropriate sedation depth is the use of bispectral index monitoring (BIS) during DISE. BIS is a modified EEG system that produces a range of values that largely correspond to a patient's state of alertness during anaesthesia.[17] It adds further information to facilitate appropriate titration of anesthetic agents in order to maintain optimal sedation levels, and recent publications suggest its use in DISE is increasing.

The role of having a data fusion system has also been described, where real-time endoscopic images of the patient's upper airways are displayed alongside the standard cardiorespiratory data from the anesthetic machine.[18] This enables both the anesthetists and surgeons to have a

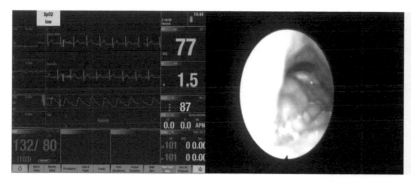

Fig. 2.1 Example of data fusion: Simultaneous cardiovascular parameters and anatomical view during drug-induced sleep endoscopy (DISE).

combined view of the airway in conjunction with the cardiovascular parameters which may lend further insight into the maintenance of optimal sedation (▶ Fig. 2.1). Interestingly, some studies have highlighted the feasibility of DISE without a dedicated anesthetist, but our own research team have no experience regarding this.[19]

2.3 Interpretation–Grading

Another great challenge of endoscopic evaluation of sleep involves establishing a consistent interpretation and means of reporting the findings. The need for consistency in reporting the findings is clear but how has it been achieved?

Croft and Pringle's published work at the Royal National Throat Nose and Ear hospital around the turn of the 1990's was the first to detail key anatomical patterns of upper airway obstruction during sedation. They were able to demonstrate in their 1991 paper how fiber optic assessment in partially anesthetized patients could convey more information about airway obstruction than clinical assessment with Müller's technique in awake SDB patients alone.[4] This article, along with Croft et al similar 1989 article about OSA in pediatric patients, were among the first to make detailed treatment recommendations based on which patterns of anatomical obstruction were observed.

The 1993 Croft and Pringle system was the first truly recognized DISE grading system and over the subsequent 25 years that have followed at least a further 15 grading systems have been published, seven of which have been named, including the more recent 2017 Kotecha–Lechner-modified Croft and Pringle system.[7] Most contemporary grading systems feature not only assessment of the patterns of upper airway obstruction but also if these patterns change with performing maneuvers that replicate the actions of sleep adjuncts such as chin straps and mandibular advancement devices, as demonstrated in ▶ Fig. 2.2 and ▶ Fig. 2.3. It was almost 2 decades after the Croft and Pringle grading system that other grading systems were proposed and amongst these are the VOTE and the NOHL classifications.[20,21]

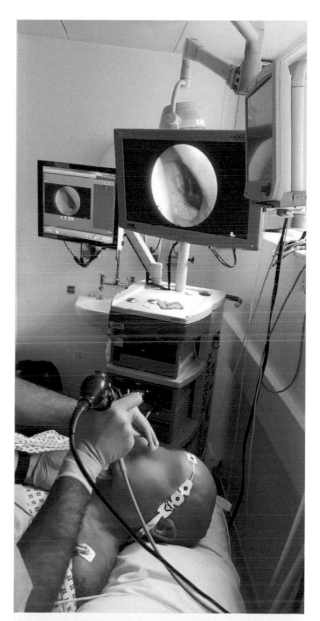

Fig. 2.2 Mouth closure and use of BIS index monitoring during DISE. Abbreviations: BIS, bispectral; DISE, drug-induced sleep endoscopy.

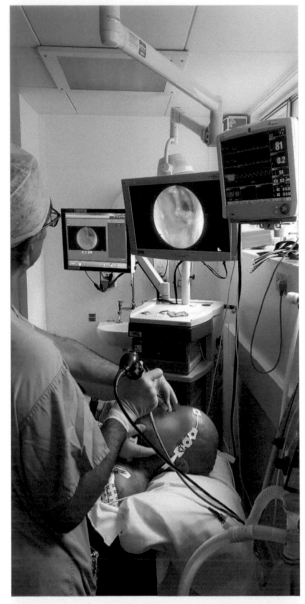

Fig. 2.3 Jaw thrust and use of BIS index monitoring during DISE. Abbreviations: BIS, bispectral; DISE, drug-induced sleep endoscopy.

2.4 Evolving Technology

Assessment during DISE started out with flexible fiber optic endoscopy via a standard eyepiece which gave the principal assessor a good appreciation of the natural tissues of the upper airways. Reproducing the image on screen has been recognized as increasingly advantageous, as it allows other members of the operating team, such as anesthetists, to also observe the patients' airway during spontaneous ventilation, potentially enabling quicker responses to maintain optimal sedation levels. This has

become increasingly feasible as technology continues to produce higher resolution cameras for traditional fiber optic scopes as well as the emergence of high-resolution flexible videoscopes that are able to capture increasingly detailed images, alongside monitors that produce increasingly clearer resolution, including the move towards ultra-high definition screens. Recording these findings may become increasingly commonplace in the future. In order to overcome the debate about comparing natural physiological sleep versus natural sleep, there have been reports of simultaneous polygraphic data being looked at during DISE.[22]

References

[1] Borowiecki B, Pollak CP, Weitzman ED, Rakoff S, Imperato J. Fibro-optic study of pharyngeal airway during sleep in patients with hypersomnia obstructive sleep-apnea syndrome. Laryngoscope. 1978; 88(8 Pt 1):1310–1313

[2] Rojewski TE, Schuller DE, Clark RW, Schmidt HS, Potts RE. Videoendoscopic determination of the mechanism of obstruction in obstructive sleep apnea. Otolaryngol Head Neck Surg. 1984; 92(2):127–131

[3] Croft CB, Thomson HG, Samuels MP, Southall DP. Endoscopic evaluation and treatment of sleep-associated upper airway obstruction in infants and young children. Clin Otolaryngol Allied Sci. 1990; 15(3):209–216

[4] Pringle MB, Croft CB. A comparison of sleep nasendoscopy and the Müller manoeuvre. Clin Otolaryngol Allied Sci. 1991; 16(6):559–562

[5] Pringle MB, Croft CB. A grading system for patients with obstructive sleep apnoea–based on sleep nasendoscopy. Clin Otolaryngol Allied Sci. 1993; 18(6):480–484

[6] De Vito A, Carrasco Llatas M, Vanni A, et al. European position paper on drug-induced sedation endoscopy (DISE). Sleep Breath. 2014; 18 (3):453–465

[7] Lechner M, Wilkins D, Kotecha B. A review on drug-induced sedation endoscopy: technique, grading systems and controversies. Sleep Med Rev. 2018; 41:141–148

[8] Kotecha BT, Hannan SA, Khalil HM, Georgalas C, Bailey P. Sleep nasendoscopy: a 10-year retrospective audit study. Eur Arch Otorhinolaryngol. 2007; 264(11):1361–1367

[9] Hewitt RJ, Dasgupta A, Singh A, Dutta C, Kotecha BT. Is sleep nasendoscopy a valuable adjunct to clinical examination in the evaluation of upper airway obstruction? Eur Arch Otorhinolaryngol. 2009; 266(5):691–697

[10] Kotecha B, De Vito A. Drug-induced sleep endoscopy: its role in evaluation of the upper airway obstruction and patient selection for surgical and non-surgical treatment. J Thorac Dis. 2018; 10 Suppl 1:S40–S47

[11] Gregório MG, Jacomelli M, Inoue D, Genta PR, de Figueiredo AC, Lorenzi-Filho G. Comparison of full versus short induced-sleep polysomnography for the diagnosis of sleep apnea. Laryngoscope. 2011; 121(5):1098–1103

[12] Abdullah VJ, Lee DLY, Ha SCN, van Hasselt CA. Sleep endoscopy with midazolam: sedation level evaluation with bispectral analysis. Otolaryngol Head Neck Surg. 2013; 148(2):331–337

[13] Marais J. The value of sedation nasendoscopy: a comparison between snoring and non-snoring patients. Clin Otolaryngol Allied Sci. 1998; 23(1):74–76

[14] Certal VF, Pratas R, Guimarães L, et al. awake examination versus DISE for surgical decision making in patients with OSA: a systematic review. Laryngoscope. 2016; 126(3):768–774

[15] Bryson HM, Fulton BR, Faulds D. Propofol. An update of its use in anaesthesia and conscious sedation. Drugs. 1995; 50(3):513–559

[16] Atkins JH, Mandel JE, Rosanova G. Safety and efficacy of drug-induced sleep endoscopy using a probability ramp propofol infusion system

in patients with severe obstructive sleep apnea. Anesth Analg. 2014; 119(4):805–810

[17] Babar-Craig H, Rajani NK, Bailey P, Kotecha BT. Validation of sleep nasendoscopy for assessment of snoring with bispectral index monitoring. Eur Arch Otorhinolaryngol. 2012; 269(4):1277–1279

[18] Dijemeni E, Kotecha B. Drug-induced sedsation endoscopy (DISE) DATA FUSION system: clinical feasibility study. Eur Arch Otorhinolaryngol. 2018; 275(1):247–260

[19] Kirkegaard Kiaer E, Tonnesen P, Sorensen HB, et al. Propofol sedation in drug induced sedation endoscopy without an anaesthesiologist: a study of safety and feasibility. Rhinology. 2019; 57(2):125–131

[20] Kezirian EJ, Hohenhorst W, de Vries N. Drug-induced sleep endoscopy: the VOTE classification. Eur Arch Otorhinolaryngol. 2011; 268(8): 1233–1236

[21] Vicini C, De Vito A, Benazzo M, et al. The nose oropharynx hypopharynx and larynx (NOHL) classification: a new system of diagnostic standardized examination for OSAHS patients. Eur Arch Otorhinolaryngol. 2012; 269(4):1297–1300

[22] Gobbi R, Baiardi S, Mondini S, et al. Technique and preliminary analysis of drug-induced sleep endoscopy with online polygraphic cardiorespiratory monitoring in patients with obstructive sleep apnea syndrome. JAMA Otolaryngol Head Neck Surg. 2017; 143(5):459–465

3 Applicability

Marina Carrasco Llatas

Abstract

Drug-induced sleep endoscopy (DISE) has emerged as the preferred tool to study the upper airway (UA) of patients with snoring or/and sleep apnea problems, as it allows the visualization of the UA in a state similar to natural sleep. In this chapter, the evidence that supports the validity of DISE will be discussed. Several articles have shown that the characteristics of the UA do not differ under sedation, as the critical closing pressure, obstruction sites, and other parameters are equivalent as long as the sedation is carefully performed. Moreover, snoring cannot be reproduced in nonsnoring patients. Summarizing, DISE is a useful tool to study the UA as it represents natural sleep.

Keywords: validity, Pcrit, BIS, drugs, natural sleep, sedation

3.1 Introduction

The main problem with upper airway (UA) examination of patients with obstructive sleep apnea (OSA) is that the easiest way to assess it is during wakefulness. The main problem is that the UA remains open without obstructions or snoring, when the patient is awake due to muscle tension. Accordingly, the pathophysiology mechanisms of the obstructions cannot be detected.

The ideal situation would be the observation of the UA during natural sleep, which is challenging in a clinical setting. This is the reason why the observation of the UA during sedation is so appealing. It offers the possibility of examining the UA during sleep and helps to detect the origins of snoring and obstructions which are causing the respiratory events during night.

Drug-induced sleep endoscopy (DISE) is a diagnostic tool. Therefore, it must match all the important characteristics required of a diagnostic tool: safety, reliability, and validity.

Since the first publication in 1991,[1] DISE has been used increasingly more worldwide as a screening tool before surgery for OSA. Nowadays, there is no doubt that the technique is safe as long as the rules for sedation are followed. DISE should be performed in a controlled and quiet room where all the anesthetic and resuscitation kits are present.[2]

Validity is the state or quality of being valid; something is valid if it is well-founded. Since the idea of DISE is to observe the UA during sleep, in order to be valid, it must represent natural sleep. Consequently, DISE should not induce snoring to control patients, and the parameters of the UA such as critical closing pressure (Pcrit) and muscle control imply that DISE should be equivalent to those obtained during natural sleep. The literature, which is supporting that DISE represents natural sleep, is discussed in this chapter.

3.2 Comparisons of Natural Sleep and Sedation

There are some studies available, comparing natural sleep and sedation with different drugs for DISE in the same people. Although the sample size of these studies is not high, the population includes obstructive sleep apnea syndrome (OSAS) patients and controls, which represent the spectrum of people who may have indications to perform DISE.

In ▶ Table 3.1, there is a brief summary of all these studies.

3.2.1 Respiratory Parameters

The first study that compared natural sleep and sedation in simple snorers and OSAS patients was conducted in Japan by Sadaoka et al in 1996.[3] They studied 50 patients comparing polysomnography (PSG) parameters obtained during natural sleep and under sedation with diazepam, which was performed during the same week. The apnea index (AI), as well as the oxygen desaturation index (ODI) and minimum oxygen saturation were equivalent in both explorations; however, with regard to the sleep structure, there was a decrease in rapid eye movement (REM) sleep as a side effect of benzodiazepine.[4]

Probably the most known study is the one made by Rabelo et al.[5] A polysomnogram (PSG) was performed for 90 to 120 minutes of sedation with propofol by using a target-controlled infusion pump (TCI) in 24 OSA patients. Thereafter, the results were compared with natural sleep. The study revealed that there were no differences in apnea–hypopnea index (AHI) or ODI. Minimum oxygen saturation was lower with sedation. Slow-wave sleep (N3) was increased and no REM sleep could be detected. Their conclusion was that the respiratory parameters did not change significantly; therefore, DISE was useful in representing natural sleep. In addition, four healthy control patients were studied, and no one snored.

Another article by Gregório et al[6] studied 25 OSAS and 15 controls sedated with midazolam comparing AHI, type of apneas (central or obstructive), and minimum oxygen saturation. They found an excellent correlation between both explorations, concluding that sedation reliably represented N1 and N2 sleep.

Table 3.1 Main characteristics of the studies comparing natural sleep and sedation

Author	N	Drug for sedation	Parameters studied	Results
Abdullah[7]	43 OSAS	Midazolam	AHI, ODI, min O_2 sat, BIS, EMG, SP	Same respiratory values, only N2 sleep during sedation. No difference in muscle relaxation
Genta[8]	15 OSAS	Midazolam	AHI, ODI, min O_2 sat, Pcrit, SP	Same respiratory values, same Pcrit, REM sleep after 90 min
Gregório[6]	25 OSAS 15 controls	Midazolam	AHI, min O_2 sat, apnea type	Same respiratory values, same apnea type No snoring in controls
Hoshino[9]	9 controls	TCI Propofol	Active and passive Pcrit, EMG, BIS	No significant difference
Morrison[10]	14 OSAS	Diazepam	Pcrit, obstruction sites	Same Pcrit and obstruction sites
Rabelo[5]	24 OSAS 4 controls	TCI Propofol	AHI, ODI, min O_2 sat, SP	Same AHI and ODI, lower min O_2 sat with sedation, increased N3, no REM No snoring in controls
Sadaoka[3]	50 SDB	Diazepam	AI, ODI, min O_2 sat, SP	Same respiratory values, less REM during sedation

Abbreviations: AI, apnea index; AHI, apnea–hypopnea index; BIS, bispectral index; Pcrit, critical closing pressure; EMG, electromyography; ODI, oxygen desaturation index; SP, sleep phases; OSAS, obstructive sleep apnea syndrome; REM, rapid eye movement.

The study by Abdullah et al[7] also confirmed that sedation represents natural sleep. As in the rest of the studies, they performed PSG and analyzed sleep phases, AHI, ODI, and minimum oxygen saturation. The innovation employed in this study was the use of bispectral index (BIS) and chin electromyography (EMG). The sample included 43 OSAS patients whose respective parameters were compared, which were obtained during midazolam sedation for 15 minutes, while the obstructions of the UA were evaluated. There was no difference in AHI, minimum oxygen saturation, and ODI. Chin EMG revealed that the muscle relaxation observed during sedation was not higher than the one in natural sleep. Moreover, BIS values were similar in both explorations in the same sleep stages. The main sleep phase observed for 15 minutes sedation was N2; therefore, their conclusion was that DISE represents N2 sleep, in which most of the respiratory events occur during the night in a vast majority of OSAS patients.

3.2.2 Critical Closing Pressure

Other studies have focused on Pcrit in order to know if sedation represents natural sleep. Pcrit can be considered as a measure of UA collapsibility and varies along a continuum from health (low collapsibility) to disease (high collapsibility).

Genta et al[8] compared 15 OSA patients in their study, wherein sedation was obtained with midazolam bolus. The findings were that there were no changes in Pcrit under sedation and obtaining REM sleep after 90 minutes.

Their conclusion was that OSA patients could be studied under sedation without bias.

Although there are differences between patients with and without OSA related to the obstruction of the UA during sleep, the studies that compare natural sleep and sedation in control patients are applicable to the issue of validity. Passive Pcrit and active Pcrit were studied in patients without sleep breathing disorders (SBDs) and the results were no different from natural sleep.[9] The compensatory responses in UA and timing parameters were well-preserved; therefore, it is likely that the collapsibility of the hypotonic pharynx is similar during sedation to that observed during natural non-REM sleep. The sedation method in the study was a TCI propofol pump.

Morrison et al[10] also focused on Pcrit of OSA patients sedated by diazepam, but they also observed the obstructions with an endoscope in 10 patients. Regarding Pcrit, an excellent correlation (r = 0.96) between natural sleep and sedation was found; furthermore, the site and degree of narrowing observed in natural sleep corresponded to those observed in diazepam-induced sleep for 15 out of 16 sites of narrowing. The difference was caused by the tongue, which moved slightly more in one patient, changing the degree of the obstruction. The excellent correlation of Pcrit and of the obstructions proved DISE as an excellent method to observe the UA.

In summary, the studies performed in 185 people comparing natural sleep and sedation concluded that sedation mimics natural sleep in non-REM sleep; therefore, DISE seems a valid tool to watch the UA of OSAS patients. For patients who only have apneas in REM sleep, DISE does not appear to be the best tool, due to the fact that REM was not possible to achieve with propofol and was observed only after 90 minutes when the sedation was performed with midazolam. At the present time, nobody knows for certain if the vibrations and obstructions observed in DISE represent those that occur during REM sleep.

3.2.3 Other Variables

It is already been explained that BIS values were equivalent in natural sleep and sedation in the same population.[7] Another study confirmed this finding using two OSA populations (one sedated population and another was studied during natural sleep), with PSG and BIS showing identical results.[11]

The recent articles focus on the nasal flow shape, as some of them are typical of specific collapses.[12,13,14] The inspiratory negative effort dependence (NED) is also a reflection of the structure that causes the UA collapse.[12,13] In May 2018, a thesis was presented comparing natural sleep and DISE with TCI-propofol, which studied these new parameters and the obstructions watched directly in both explorations.[15] The correlation of the endoscopic results was strong for the tongue, substantial for the velum and epiglottis, and moderate for the oropharynx. The NED evaluations revealed a similar collapsibility in both situations. Propofol did not impair the respiratory drive. The conclusion of the study was that the use of propofol during DISE had no effect on the UA collapsibility when compared to sleep endoscopy during natural sleep.

3.3 DISE Validity and Sedation Method

The results of the studies mentioned before endorse the idea that DISE represents natural sleep; nevertheless, there are articles that affirm that DISE is not reliable because it can reproduce snoring in nonsnoring patients or create excessive tongue obstructions.[16,17] The different sedation methods and drugs used for sedation may be responsible for this issue. Although the anesthetic aspects of DISE and drugs will be discussed in Chapter 9 and Chapter 10, it is important to summarize some studies in this chapter.

There are few articles that compare the UA of the same patients sedated by two different drugs, with two of them comparing propofol and dexmedetomidine. These studies state that there are no important differences in the UA obstruction when the sedation level is the same.[18,19] In a deeper sedation, the obstruction is increased similarly with both drugs.[18] One article compared propofol and midazolam and found no important differences in UA collapse or AHI[20]. Another study focusing on comparing propofol and midazolam concluded that Pcrit was identical

for each patient with both drugs, but different among patients,[21] representing the diverse Pcrit in different people but being constant for an individual.

One may think that what sedation drug is used or how it is delivered to perform DISE does not matter, but this is not true. The patient must have the exact level of sedation; if it is light, there will not be obstructions or snoring, and if it is too deep, the UA will show fake obstructions caused by the sedative drug.[22,23,24] Therefore, it is recommended to monitor the level of sedation using BIS or another analogue device, with the right level usually being in the range from 75 to 50, although there is interindividual variability, so this may not apply to everyone. Although BIS values around 40 are the ones observed during N3 sleep, most of the obstructions occur in N2. There is no need to achieve a deeper sedation that may lead to a fake UA collapse. Furthermore, another study revealed that there was a change of treatment plan when patients passed from light to moderate sedation (BIS values from 80 to 60), but the strategy did not change once the sedation deepened from 60 to 50.[23]

If the drug used for sedation is propofol, it is strongly recommended to deliver the drug using a TCI pump, as the bolus technique can produce oversedation and lower desaturations; moreover, UA behavior is not reliable, leading to wrong therapeutic decisions.[25,26] Moreover, snoring can be reproduced in all OSA patients with the TCI-propofol technique (by slowly increasing the drug concentration) but it was not observed in any of the 54 controls despite high brain concentrations of 8 µg/mL, which triplicate the usual starting dose concentration.[27]

In brief, the studies that have been conducted comparing natural sleep and sedation support the validity of DISE. DISE is a useful tool to study the UA, as it represents no REM sleep, specially N1 and N2 phases. Apparently, this is true no matter what drug is used for sedation (diazepam, midazolam, propofol, or dexmedetomidine). Nevertheless, the validity of propofol has only been proven when it is delivered using a TCI pump, therefore propofol should be preferably administrated with this method.

References

[1] Croft CB, Pringle M. Sleep nasendoscopy: a technique of assessment in snoring and obstructive sleep apnoea. Clin Otolaryngol Allied Sci. 1991; 16(5):504–509

[2] De Vito A, Carrasco Llatas M, Vanni A, et al. European position paper on drug-induced sedation endoscopy (DISE). Sleep Breath. 2014; 18 (3):453–465

[3] Sadaoka T, Kakitsuba N, Fujiwara Y, Kanai R, Takahashi H. The value of sleep nasendoscopy in the evaluation of patients with suspected sleep-related breathing disorders. Clin Otolaryngol Allied Sci. 1996; 21(6):485–489

[4] Pagel JF, Parnes BL. Medications for the treatment of sleep disorders: an overview. Prim Care Companion J Clin Psychiatry. 2001; 3(3): 118–125

[5] Rabelo FAW, Küpper DS, Sander HH, Fernandes RMF, Valera FCP. Polysomnographic evaluation of propofol-induced sleep in patients with

respiratory sleep disorders and controls. Laryngoscope. 2013; 123 (9):2300–2305

[6] Gregório MG, Jacomelli M, Inoue D, Genta PR, de Figueiredo AC, Lorenzi-Filho G. Comparison of full versus short induced-sleep polysomnography for the diagnosis of sleep apnea. Laryngoscope. 2011; 121(5):1098–1103

[7] Abdullah VJ, Lee DLY, Ha SCN, van Hasselt CA. Sleep endoscopy with midazolam: sedation level evaluation with bispectral analysis. Otolaryngol Head Neck Surg. 2013; 148(2):331–337

[8] Genta PR, Eckert DJ, Gregório MG, et al. Critical closing pressure during midazolam-induced sleep. J Appl Physiol (1985). 2011; 111 (5):1315–1322

[9] Hoshino Y, Ayuse T, Kurata S, et al. The compensatory responses to upper airway obstruction in normal subjects under propofol anesthesia. Respir Physiol Neurobiol. 2009; 166(1):24–31

[10] Morrison DL, Launois SH, Isono S, Feroah TR, Whitelaw WA, Remmers JE. Pharyngeal narrowing and closing pressures in patients with obstructive sleep apnea. Am Rev Respir Dis. 1993; 148(3):606–611

[11] Babar-Craig H, Rajani NK, Bailey P, Kotecha BT. Validation of sleep nasendoscopy for assessment of snoring with bispectral index monitoring. Eur Arch Otorhinolaryngol. 2012; 269(4): 1277–1279

[12] Genta PR, Sands SA, Butler JP, et al. Airflow shape is associated with the pharyngeal structure causing OSA. Chest. 2017; 152(3):537–546

[13] Azarbarzin A, Sands SA, Marques M, et al. Palatal prolapse as a signature of expiratory flow limitation and inspiratory palatal collapse in patients with obstructive sleep apnoea. Eur Respir J. 2018; 51(2): 1701419

[14] Marques M, Genta PR, Azarbarzin A, et al. Retropalatal and retroglossal airway compliance in patients with obstructive sleep apnea. Respir Physiol Neurobiol. 2018; 258(June):98–103

[15] Ordones AB. Sonoendoscopia durante sono natural comparada com sonoendoscopia durante sono induzido com propofol. Available at: http://www.teses.usp.br/teses/disponiveis/5/5143/tde-15082018-105521/. Accessed August 29, 2018

[16] El Badawey MR, McKee G, Heggie N, Marshall H, Wilson JA. Predictive value of sleep nasendoscopy in the management of habitual snorers. Ann Otol Rhinol Laryngol. 2003; 112(1):40–44

[17] Capasso R, Rosa T, Tsou DY-A, et al. Variable findings for drug-induced sleep endoscopy in obstructive sleep apnea with propofol versus dexmedetomidine. Otolaryngol Head Neck Surg. 2016; 154(4):765–770

[18] Yoon B-W, Hong J-M, Hong S-L, Koo S-K, Roh H-J, Cho K-S. A comparison of dexmedetomidine versus propofol during drug-induced sleep endoscopy in sleep apnea patients. Laryngoscope. 2016; 126(3):763–767

[19] Mahmoud M, Gunter J, Donnelly LF, Wang Y, Nick TG, Sadhasivam S. A comparison of dexmedetomidine with propofol for magnetic resonance imaging sleep studies in children. Anesth Analg. 2009; 109(3): 745–753

[20] Carrasco Llatas M, Agostini Porras G, Cuesta González MT, et al. Drug-induced sleep endoscopy: a two drug comparison and simultaneous polysomnography. Eur Arch Otorhinolaryngol. 2014; 271(1):181–187

[21] Norton JR, Ward DS, Karan S, et al. Differences between midazolam and propofol sedation on upper airway collapsibility using dynamic negative airway pressure. Anesthesiology. 2006; 104(6):1155–1164

[22] Kellner P, Herzog B, Plößl S, et al. Depth-dependent changes of obstruction patterns under increasing sedation during drug-induced sedation endoscopy: results of a German monocentric clinical trial. Sleep Breath. 2016; 20(3):1035–1043

[23] Heiser C, Fthenakis P, Hapfelmeier A, et al. Drug-induced sleep endoscopy with target-controlled infusion using propofol and monitored depth of sedation to determine treatment strategies in obstructive sleep apnea. Sleep Breath. 2017; 21(3):737–744

[24] Hong SD, Dhong H-J, Kim HY, et al. Change of obstruction level during drug-induced sleep endoscopy according to sedation depth in obstructive sleep apnea. Laryngoscope. 2013; 123(11):2896–2899

[25] De Vito A, Agnoletti V, Berrettini S, et al. Drug-induced sleep endoscopy: conventional versus target controlled infusion techniques—a randomized controlled study. Eur Arch Otorhinolaryngol. 2011; 268 (3):457–462

[26] De Vito A, Agnoletti V, Zani G, et al. The importance of drug-induced sedation endoscopy (DISE) techniques in surgical decision-making: conventional versus target controlled infusion techniques—a prospective randomized controlled study and a retrospective surgical outcomes analysis. Eur Arch Otorhinolaryngol. 2017; 274(5):2307–2317

[27] Berry S, Roblin G, Williams A, Watkins A, Whittet HB. Validity of sleep nasendoscopy in the investigation of sleep related breathing disorders. Laryngoscope. 2005; 115(3):538–540

4 Classifications Systems

Marina Carrasco Llatas

Abstract

Through the last few decades, many different drug-induced sleep endoscopy (DISE) classification systems have been proposed. These vary from very complex and over comprehensive to very simple. This chapter provides an overview of the different systems and discusses the advantages and disadvantages of the most used classification systems.

Keywords: obstructive sleep apnea, drug-induced sleep endoscopy, classification

4.1 Introduction

Drug-induced sleep endoscopy (DISE) is a unique diagnostic technique that allows the direct visualization of the upper airway (UA) of snorers or obstructive sleep apnea (OSA) patients under a condition that simulates natural sleep. Introduced in 1991 by Croft and Pringle,[1] DISE has gain popularity among ENTs all over the world, because the complexity of the mechanisms of the obstruction at the different areas of the UA can be observed during DISE. Therefore, a tailor-made treatment can be offered to patients.

The initial grading scale used by Pringle and Croft was a simple system evaluating the location of obstruction only at the velopharyngeal level, oropharyngeal level, or both. Nowadays, more than 20 classification systems coexist in the literature.[2] This is the reflection of the complexity of the anatomy of the UA and a consequence of the historical evolution of DISE and surgical techniques. Furthermore, the knowledge acquired with the UA visualization has highlighted that simple classifications did not pay adequate attention to a pivotal element of the UA: the lateral pharyngeal walls (LPW) and how their movement can affect the collapse. Besides, the initial classification systems were designed to identify ideal adult candidates for uvulopalatopharyngoplasty (UPPP), with the goal of improving the success rate for this procedure. Nevertheless, since that time, a number of additional surgical treatment options have been developed for obstructive sleep apnea (OSA), which require a scoring system that considers additional sites of pharyngeal and laryngeal obstruction and potential treatment options.

The coexistence of so many classification systems is a serious limitation of DISE in order to compare the different obstruction patterns among patients and centers but maybe it is not so important in order to plan the above-mentioned tailor-made treatment. In the updated European position paper on DISE,[3] a recommended report is suggested, in which a brief explanation of the vibrations and obstructions and how they change with the different maneuvers should be written. In fact, it has been published that many ENT who perform DISE in the UK do not use a specific classification, and they just write down what they observed during the exploration.[4]

Despite this fact, the use of a classification system allows comparison of the type of collapse and the surgical outcomes in order to know if one surgical technique is better than another to treat one specific type of collapse. Using a common classification also would allow learning from other teams' experience regarding oral appliances, etc. In this chapter, the main classification systems that have been published will be reviewed.

4.2 Anatomy

The physicians who perform DISE are well-aware of the anatomy of the UA, nevertheless it is important to remind some basic ideas. The tumor/node/metastasis (TNM) classification for tumors of the American Joint Committee on Cancer (AJCC) provides a common language to all the physicians who treat the UA.[5] According to it, the UA is organized into several major sites that are subdivided into several anatomic subsites. The major sites that can be involved in a collapse include the oropharynx, hypopharynx, larynx, nasopharynx, and nose. The nose cannot cause a dynamic collapse, therefore it is not important for DISE. The oropharynx begins where the oral cavity ends at the junction of the hard and soft palates superiorly and the circumvallate papillae inferiorly and extends from the level of the soft palate superiorly, which separates it from the nasopharynx, to the level of the hyoid bone inferiorly. The subsites of the oropharynx are the tonsil, base of tongue, soft palate, and pharyngeal walls. The hypopharynx has its superior limit at the level of the hyoid bone, and extends inferiorly to the cricopharyngeus muscle, as it transitions to the cervical esophagus. Due to its caudal location, the hypopharynx does not play a major role in the obstruction of the UA in most of the patients. Accordingly, saying hypopharyngeal collapse to the collapse located at the tongue base, as the tongue base belongs to the oropharynx, should be avoided (▶ Fig. 4.1).

Another important issue is the overlap of the structures in the oropharynx, which is important, especially between the soft palate and the upper part of the tongue base. During the awake exploration of the mouth and oropharynx in many OSA patients, it is not possible to see the lower part of the palate or the posterior wall even though the mouth is open and the tongue is depressed. It is easy to imagine that when we look at the UA from the nasopharynx with the endoscope, the soft

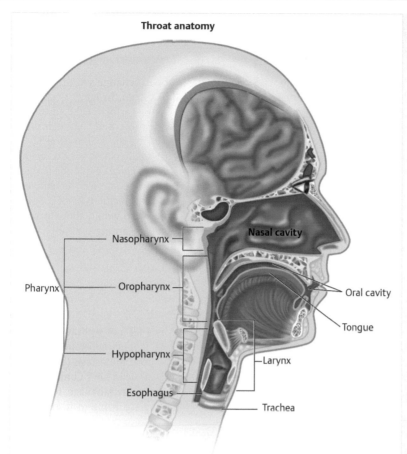

Throat anatomy

Nasopharynx

Pharynx

Oropharynx

Hypopharynx

Esophagus

Nasal cavity

Oral cavity

Tongue

Larynx

Trachea

Fig. 4.1 Drawing of the UA and the sites/subsites. Abbreviation: UA, upper airway.

palate will cover the upper part of the tongue base, and when one sees clearly the tongue, it is the lower part of the tongue base what is observed.

During DISE, it is important to remember this situation, as it is possible that a collapse observed in the velopharyngeal region is actually caused by the upper part of the tongue base which falls backward, pushing the soft palate against the posterior wall (causing a secondary palatal collapse). This is more frequently observed if the patient has the mouth open. The lower part of the tongue base is where the lingual tonsils are located and may contribute to the obstruction, being the main cause of collapse in some patients. It is important to notice that the collapse could be due to a lymphoid tissue hypertrophy or an anteroposterior collapse by the muscle itself, as the surgical plan will be different: if the lymphoid tissue is hypertrophic, a lingual tonsillectomy could be successful, but if it is a collapse caused by the muscle itself, hypoglossal nerve stimulation could prove to be the best choice.

Palatine tonsils are located in the LPW and contribute to the lateral collapse when they are present. During DISE, it can be easy to visualize this collapse when tonsils are big. Otherwise, when they are small, it can be difficult to distinguish from a previous tonsillectomized patient.

4.3 Main Elements that a DISE Scoring System Should Have

Although there is no consensus on a unique classification system, the working group of the European position paper on DISE reached a general agreement on the elements that any classification should have. The scoring and classification system should include the following features: level (and/or structure), degree (severity), and configuration (pattern and direction) of obstruction.[6]

Regarding the number of levels, some presently used systems identify four levels of obstruction, while others distinguish five levels. Some systems use levels, others prefer structures, while others, for pragmatic reasons, use a hybrid system, including both levels and structures.

Some systems have only three degrees of severity (none, partial, and complete obstruction), whereas other systems use a semiquantitative system with 0–25, 25–50, 50–75, and 75–100% of obstruction. By using the second system, it is easier to make comparisons between awake exploration and DISE, because this is how the Müller maneuver is rated, although it has a disadvantage because more degrees of obstruction decrease interrater reliability.

In the pediatric population, the existence of hypertrophic adenoid tissue makes the assessment of obstruction at the nasopharyngeal level absolutely necessary, whereas in adults, obstruction at this level is uncommon, and this is the reason why many classification systems for adults do not report nasopharyngeal analysis.

4.4 Common Classification Systems

4.4.1 Pringle and Croft

The first classification was published in 1993. It divides patients into five groups (▶ Table 4.1). This system does not pay attention to the shape of the collapse or the epiglottic collapse. The degree of collapse is not clearly defined either and may not be intuitive.

Kotecha and Lechner have recently published an update[8] for this classification, in which they specify the shape and the configuration of the collapse and include epiglottic collapse within grade V (▶ Table 4.2).[7]

Table 4.1 Pringle and Croft DISE classification

Grade 1	Simple palatal snoring
Grade 2	Single level palatal obstruction
Grade 3	Multisegmental involvement: intermittent orohypopharyngeal collapse
Grade 4	Sustained multisegmental collapse
Grade 5	Tongue base collapse

Abbreviation: DISE, drug-induced sedation endoscopy.

4.4.2 The VOTE Classification

VOTE is an acronym for velum, oropharynx, tongue base, and epiglottis. This classification is simple and intuitive. It considers the structure causing the collapse, as well as the degree of collapse (none, partial or complete) and its configuration (anteroposterior, lateral, or concentric; ▶ Table 4.3).[9] To our knowledge, it is the most frequently used in the literature, because of its simplicity.[2] Nevertheless, it does not pay attention to the nose or nasopharynx, diminishing its use for the pediatric population. Moreover, at the tongue base level, the only possible configuration is anteroposterior. Although this is the most frequent configuration of the collapse observed in this area, in some patients, the pattern can be circular due to the contribution of the LPW to the collapse; in a few patients, the tongue can bend like a book, creating a lateral collapse. This is the reason why some authors modified this classification, allowing the possibility to have lateral or concentric collapse in this area too,[10] and the European working group recommended the use of this classification as it is in ▶ Table 4.3, allowing all kind of configurations at the tongue base. The VOTE classification does not have a specific level for other laryngeal structures which may cause obstruction in few patients such as the ariepiglottic folds; nevertheless, it can be written as an addendum in case it is necessary.

4.4.3 The NOHL Classification

Introduced by Vicini et al in 2012, this classification can be applied to both awake and DISE exploration. The Nose (including the nose and nasopharynx), Oropharynx (equivalent to velum in VOTE classification), Hypopharynx (equivalent to tongue base in VOTE), and Larynx (in which a supraglottic or type a, or glottic type b) are the areas where

Table 4.2 The Kotecha and Lechner classification

Grade I	Palatal flutter ☐	
Grade II	Palatal flutter + nasopharyngeal collapse ☐ AP ☐ Lateral ☐ Concentric	

Grade III	Multisegmental collapse on inspiration	• Nasopharynx..........%
		• Oropharynx............%
		   ☐ Lateral wall collapse
		   ☐ AP collapse
		   ☐ Circumferential collapse
		• Tongue base............%

Grade IV	Multisegmental (on inspiration/expiration) ☐	
Grade V	Tongue base + /− epiglottic retraction ☐	

Table 4.3 The VOTE classification

Structure	Degree of obstruction	Configuration		
		Anteroposterior	Lateral	Concentric
Velum				
Oropharynx				
Tongue base				
Epiglottis				

0: No obstruction.
1: Partial obstruction (vibration).
2: Complete obstruction (collapse > 75%).
X: Not visualized.

Table 4.4 The NOHL classification

Site	Nose static obstruction	Oropharynx	Hypopharynx	Larynx a: supraglottic b: glottic
Static nasal obstruction/ pharynx collapse % grade value: 1–4	0–25%: 1 25–50%: 2 50–75%: 3 75–100%: 4	0–25%: 1 25–50%: 2 50–75%: 3 75–100%: 4	0–25%: 1 25–50%: 2 50–75%: 3 75–100%: 4	Positive or negative collapse/obstruction

the collapse can be observed. The degree of the configuration can be rated from 0 to 4, and the configuration can be anteroposterior, lateral or circular. The collapse observed is written in accordance with the TNM classification. For example, N0 O4c H1ap L0 is related to a patient with a complete circular collapse at the velum with less than 25% anteroposterior obstruction at the tongue base without nose either nasopharyngeal obstruction or laryngeal obstruction. When tonsil hypertrophy causes collapse, they are added in the sentence using the letters "TS" (tonsil) (▶ Table 4.4).

This classification is easy to apply, but as explained before, the terminology hypopharynx for tongue base collapse is inaccurate and may lead to misunderstandings.[11]

4.4.4 Bachar's Classification

Also introduced in 2012 by Bachar et al (▶ Table 4.5), this classification identifies the UA sites, including the nose and nasopharynx (N), palatine plane, uvula, or tonsils (P), tongue base (T), larynx (L), and hypopharynx (H). The obstruction is categorized as partial (1) or complete (2). The configuration of the collapse is not rated. Likewise, in the NOHL classification, the UA collapse is written in a sentence mode. For example, P2 T2 E1, afterward the numbers are added, and a staging index is obtained. This staging index shared a correlation with the respiratory disturbance index (RDI). Although this classification includes all the possible areas that can cause an obstruction, and it would be useful for pediatric DISE too, it excludes the configuration of

Table 4.5 Bachar's classification

Zone	No collapse	Partial collapse	Complete collapse
Nose/nasopharynx	0	1	2
Palate (tonsils included)	0	1	2
Tongue base	0	1	2
Larynx	0	1	2
Hypopharynx	0	1	2

the collapse; therefore, it is not useful to select patients for hypoglossal nerve stimulation.[12,13]

4.4.5 Woodson's Classification

Woodson's classification is also thought to be used both in awake and DISE settings (▶ Table 4.6). Seven anatomic reference points are selected for measuring the UA lumen's cross-sectional size and shape (hard palate, genu of the soft palate, velum, velopharyngeal lateral wall, pharyngeal tongue, vallecular tongue, and epiglottis), and one soft tissue landmark: lingual tonsils. The shape of the UA is rated as 1 + when it is patent, 2 + when is narrowed, 3 + if it is compromised, and 4 + if it is obstructed.[14]

Table 4.6 Woodson's classification

UA levels	UA lumen rating scale			
	+1	+2	+3	+4
Hard palate	Patent	–	–	Obstructed
Genu of the soft palate	Patent	–	Compromised	Obstructed
Velum (anterior, posterior)	Patent	–	Compromised	Obstructed
Lateral wall (at velum)	Patent (wide)	Patent	Compromised	Obstructed
Pharyngeal tongue	Patent	Narrowed	Compromised	Obstructed
Vallecular tongue	Patent	Narrowed	Compromised	Obstructed
Epiglottis	Patent	Narrowed	Compromised	Obstructed
Lingual tonsil	Absent	Present	Enlarged	Obstructed

Abbreviation: UA, upper airway.

This classification is difficult to rate in DISE due to the constant movement of the UA; besides, as it has four grades of obstruction, the interrater agreement may be lower than when less degrees of obstruction are used.

4.4.6 Other Mixed Classifications

Gillespie et al[15] published a mixed classification in which the palatine tonsils are apart from the lateral pharyngeal walls, being an independent area, and the presence or absence of the lingual tonsil is rated different if it causes a complete or partial obstruction. Although the idea of specifying the obstruction caused by the lingual tonsil at the tongue base has an important impact on the plan of the surgical technique, unless the palatine tonsils are grade 3 or 4, it is difficult to separate their obstruction from the LPW. As with the Bachar's classification, all the obstructions can be added to create a scoring index which is related to the apnea–hypopnea index (AHI).

Koo et al[16] also use a mixed classification where the degree is rated from 0 to 2. Collapse is rated in the retropalatal and retrolingual area; the configuration (anteroposterior or lateral) and the main structure contributing to the collapse (tonsil in the retropalatal and epiglottis in the retrolingual) is also expressed. Therefore, in the retropalatal area, the concentric collapse is described when there is an anteroposterior and lateral movement.

There are more classifications published, such as the one published by Kellner et al,[17] even an attempt was made in order to unify all the different classifications into one universal scoring system.[18] Nevertheless, explaining in detail all the differences among these classifications goes beyond the scope of this chapter.

According to Amos et al,[2] the ideal grading system would include elements of the VOTE classification system[9]

Table 4.7 The Chang scoring template for pediatric sleep endoscopy

Indicate the greatest (box) and least (circle) obstructed views for each of the following locations:	
Adenoid	0 1 2 3
Velum	0 1 2 3
LPW/tonsils	0 1 2 3
Tongue base	0 1 2 3
Supraglottis	0 1 2 3
Lingual tonsils	Present/absent

Abbreviation: LPW, lateral pharyngeal walls.

and the DISE grading system published by Bachar et al.[12] The VOTE classification is simple to use and includes the direction/shape of obstruction. The Bachar system includes assessment of the nose/nasopharynx and larynx. It also includes an overall sleep index, which correlates with the respiratory disturbance index and body mass index (BMI). Both systems include two degrees of obstruction (partial and complete).

4.4.7 Pediatric Classifications

The specific pediatric characteristic of the UA made it necessary to propose a specific classification system.

Although Boudewyns et al published a classification in 2014,[19] the one published by Chan et al[20] is closer to the ones used for adults; therefore, this one is the one that will be explained (▶ Table 4.7).

For each location, assess the view obtained at the most and least obstructed points in respiratory cycle.

- *Adenoid: Posterior view from nasal cavity* (0 = absent adenoids; 1 = 0–50% obstruction of choana; 2 = 50–99% obstruction of choana; 3 = complete obstruction of choana).
- *Velum: Inferior view from nasopharynx; assessing anterior–posterior obstruction* (0 = no obstruction [complete view of tongue base and/or larynx]; 1 = 0–50% anterior–posterior closure [some view of tongue base/larynx]; 2 = 50–99% anterior-posterior closure [no view of tongue base/larynx, but not against posterior pharyngeal wall]; 3 = complete closure against posterior pharyngeal wall).
- *LPW: Inferior view from velum; assessing LPW/tonsillar obstruction* (0 = no obstruction; 1 = 0–50% lateral obstruction; 2 = 50–99% lateral obstruction; 3 = complete obstruction).
- *Tongue base: Inferior view from oropharynx; assessing anterior–posterior obstruction* (0 = no obstruction [complete view of vallecula]; 1 = 0–50% obstruction [vallecula not visible]; 2 = 50–99% obstruction [epiglottis not contacting posterior pharyngeal wall]; 3 = complete obstruction [epiglottis against posterior pharyngeal wall]).
- *Supraglottis: Inferior view with tongue base (if obstructing) out of the way, with or without jaw thrust* (0 = no obstruction (full view of vocal cords); 1 = 0–50% obstruction (vocal cords partially obscured but >50% visible); 2 = 50–99% obstruction (>50% of vocal cords obscured); 3 = complete obstruction (glottic opening not seen).

4.5 Localization of the Tip of the Endoscope

In order to score correctly. the degree and the shape of the UA collapse, and the tip of the endoscope must be located at the right position, therefore it is of upmost importance to mention these exact positions where the scoring analysis must be performed. The endoscope should be placed at the level of the choanae to assess the soft palate (i.e., velum), at the level of the caudal margin of the soft palate to assess the oropharynx, and just above the level of the tongue base to assess the tongue base and the epiglottis.

4.6 Images of Collapses

See ▶ Fig. 4.2, ▶ Fig. 4.3, ▶ Fig. 4.4, ▶ Fig. 4.5, ▶ Fig. 4.6, ▶ Fig. 4.7, and ▶ Fig. 4.8.

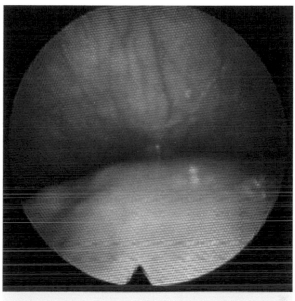

Fig. 4.2 Complete AP velum collapse. Abbreviation: AP, anteroposterior.

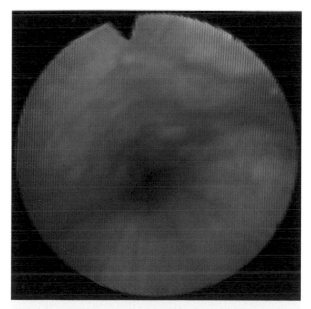

Fig. 4.3 Complete circumferential collapse at the velum.

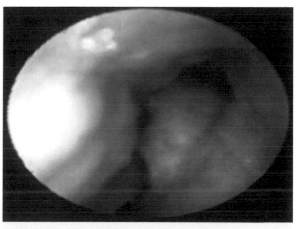

Fig. 4.4 Complete collapse due to kissing tonsils.

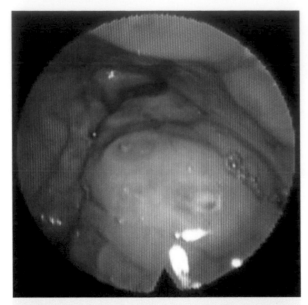

Fig. 4.5 Complete tongue base collapse due to lingual tonsils hypertrophy.

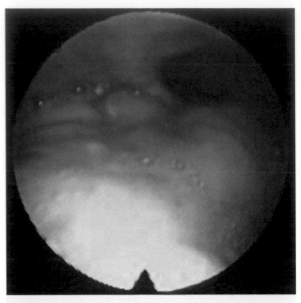

Fig. 4.6 Complete tongue base collapse without significant lingual tonsils hypertrophy.

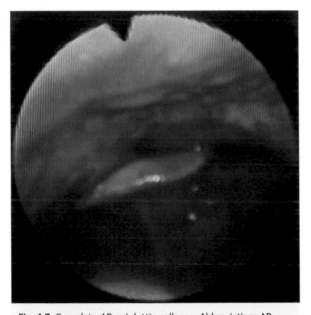

Fig. 4.7 Complete AP epiglottis collapse. Abbreviation: AP, anteroposterior.

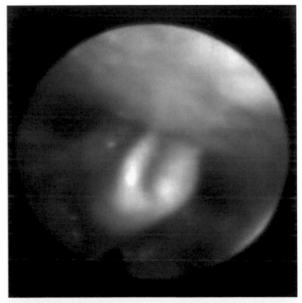

Fig. 4.8 Complete lateral epiglottis collapse.

4.7 Conclusions

There are many classification systems for DISE, reflecting the complex anatomy of the UA, personal experience of the DISE experts, and evolution of the surgical techniques available to treat OSA patients. The lack of universally accepted DISE classification is an obstacle to perform comparisons among patients and different centers. Nevertheless, DISE provides a dynamic three-dimensional (3D) UA visualization in a state that simulates sleep, which is essential for the diagnosis of the collapse and a customized treatment.

References

[1] Croft CB, Pringle M. Sleep nasendoscopy: a technique of assessment in snoring and obstructive sleep apnoea. Clin Otolaryngol Allied Sci. 1991; 16(5):504–509

[2] Amos JM, Durr ML, Nardone HC, Baldassari CM, Duggins A, Ishman SL. Systematic review of drug-induced sleep endoscopy scoring systems. Otolaryngol Head Neck Surg. 2018; 158(2):240–248

[3] De Vito A, Carrasco Llatas M, Ravesloot MJ, et al. European position paper on drug-induced sleep endoscopy: 2017 Update. Clin Otolaryngol. 2018; 43(6):1541–1552

[4] Veer V, Zhang H, Beyers J, Vanderveken O, Kotecha B. The use of drug-induced sleep endoscopy in England and Belgium. Eur Arch Otorhinolaryngol. 2018; 275(5):1335–1342

[5] Greene FL, Balch CM, Fleming ID, et al. AJCC Cancer Staging Handbook: TNM Classification of Malignant Tumors. Springer Science & Business Media; 2002

[6] De Vito A, Carrasco Llatas M, Vanni A, et al. European position paper on drug-induced sedation endoscopy (DISE). Sleep Breath. 2014; 18 (3):453–465

[7] Pringle MB, Croft CB. A grading system for patients with obstructive sleep apnoea–based on sleep nasendoscopy. Clin Otolaryngol Allied Sci. 1993; 18(6):480–484

[8] Kotecha B, Lechner M. Advancing the grading for drug-induced sleep endoscopy: a useful modification of the Croft–Pringle Grading system. Sleep Breath. 2018; 22(1):193–194

[9] Kezirian EJ, Hohenhorst W, de Vries N. Drug-induced sleep endoscopy: the VOTE classification. Eur Arch Otorhinolaryngol. 2011; 268 (8):1233–1236

[10] Carrasco-Llatas M, Zerpa-Zerpa V, Dalmau-Galofre J. Reliability of drug-induced sedation endoscopy: interobserver agreement. Sleep Breath. 2017; 21(1):173–179

[11] Vicini C, De Vito A, Benazzo M, et al. The nose oropharynx hypopharynx and larynx (NOHL) classification: a new system of diagnostic standardized examination for OSAHS patients. Eur Arch Otorhinolaryngol. 2012; 269(4):1297–1300

[12] Bachar G, Nageris B, Feinmesser R, et al. Novel grading system for quantifying upper-airway obstruction on sleep endoscopy. Lung. 2012; 190(3).313–318

[13] Vanderveken OM, Maurer JT, Hohenhorst W, et al. Evaluation of drug-induced sleep endoscopy as a patient selection tool for implanted upper airway stimulation for obstructive sleep apnea. J Clin Sleep Med. 2013; 9(5):433–438

[14] Woodson BT. A method to describe the pharyngeal airway. Laryngoscope. 2015; 125(5):1233–1238

[15] Gillespie MB, Reddy RP, White DR, Discolo CM, Overdyk FJ, Nguyen SA. A trial of drug-induced sleep endoscopy in the surgical management of sleep-disordered breathing. Laryngoscope. 2013; 123(1):277–282

[16] Koo SK, Choi JW, Myung NS, Lee HJ, Kim YJ, Kim YJ. Analysis of obstruction site in obstructive sleep apnea syndrome patients by drug induced sleep endoscopy. Am J Otolaryngol. 2013; 34(6):626–630

[17] Kellner P, Herzog B, Plößl S, et al. Depth-dependent changes of obstruction patterns under increasing sedation during drug-induced sedation endoscopy: results of a German monocentric clinical trial. Sleep Breath. 2016; 20(3):1035–1043

[18] Dijemeni E, D'Amone G, Gbati I, uDISE model: a universal drug-induced sedation endoscopy classification system-part 1. Eur Arch Otorhinolaryngol. 2017; 274(10):3795–3801

[19] Boudewyns A, Verhulst S, Maris M, Saldien V, Van de Heyning PH. Drug-induced sedation endoscopy in pediatric obstructive sleep apnea syndrome. Sleep Med. 2014; 15(12):1526–1531

[20] Chan DK, Liming BJ, Horn DL, Parikh SR. A new scoring system for upper airway pediatric sleep endoscopy. JAMA Otolaryngol Head Neck Surg. 2014; 140(7):595–602

5 Indications and Contraindications

Nico de Vries and Olivier M. Vanderveken

Abstract

An indication is a valid reason to perform a procedure or surgical intervention; a contraindication is a reason to withhold this. In this chapter, indications, contraindications, geographical differences, drug-induced sleep endoscopy (DISE) in obstructive sleep apnea (OSA) treatment of naïve patients, DISE and positional OSA, DISE in upper airway (UA) surgery and UA stimulation, DISE in simple snorers, DISE after failure of UA surgery, UA stimulation and continuous positive airway pressure (CPAP), and DISE after weight loss and persistent pathology are all discussed.

Keywords: obstructive sleep apnea, drug-induced sleep endoscopy, indications, contraindications

5.1 Introduction and Definitions

In medicine, an indication is defined as a valid reason to perform a certain test, use medication, and perform a procedure or surgical intervention. The opposite of an indication is a contraindication, a reason to withhold a certain medical treatment or procedure because the risks clearly outweigh the benefits, or that the procedure serves no purpose. There must be a good reason to perform drug-induced sleep endoscopy (DISE), and that reason is that DISE findings might influence therapeutic advice. DISE findings can indeed make the difference between nonsurgical and surgical therapy, and in case of surgery, it is important which surgical procedure(s) to perform. On the other hand, if it is already decided that a patient with sleep-disordered breathing (SDB) will undergo a certain treatment, in particular continuous positive airway pressure (CPAP), or a specific combination of treatments, one could argue that DISE might not be indicated. Another reason to perform DISE is to exclude findings that would make a certain procedure not indicated; for example, complete concentric palatal collapse being a contraindication for upper airway stimulation (UAS) therapy.[1]

The clinical reality is that DISE is mostly performed in case UA surgery is considered. Another reason for DISE is if UA stimulation is considered, since at this stage, as mentioned before, complete concentric collapse at the level of the palate level (CCCp) during DISE is a strict contraindication for UAS. In fact, the STAR trial was the first trial in which the FDA-approved DISE as a formal treatment selection tool in order for a patient with obstructive sleep apnea (OSA) to be eligible for UAS.[2] In how far DISE is useful in case of treatment with an oral device using mandibular advancement devices (MADs) or positional therapy is considered more controversial and depends on the circumstances and availability of potential alternatives. In a recent paper, however, the presence of CCCp and/or a laterolateral collapse at the level of the oropharynx are related with unsuccessful MAD treatment; while tongue base collapse during baseline DISE seems to be favorable for MAD success.[3]

5.2 Geographical Differences

There are important geographical differences that cannot be ignored. In some parts of the world, for example in North America, treatment of OSA is still very much dominated by CPAP prescribers. In many countries, reimbursement of UA surgery, UA stimulation and the diagnostic step before that—DISE—is often not available. Remarkably, there are also countries where sleep surgery is paid for, while CPAP is not. So, when we discuss indications and contraindications for DISE, the most important factor is very basal: is DISE and subsequent sleep surgery (and UAS) reimbursed or not?

At the other side of the spectrum, in other countries, many different forms of treatment are reimbursed on "good indication." The Netherlands might very well be the country in the world where the concept of treatment diversification for OSA has landed the most. Here, many forms of treatment—CPAP, MAD, positional therapy, UA surgery, UAS, and bariatric surgery—are all considered good treatment as stated in the Dutch guideline for "Diagnosis and Treatment of Obstructive Sleep Apnea in Adults." While even in the Netherlands, UA surgery and UAS are to a certain extend regarded as something that has to be avoided as much as possible, the role of DISE, in case these treatments are considered is regarded less controversial. Apparently, when surgery is considered, it is felt that it is the responsibility of the surgeon to perform as careful a workup as possible. It is a fact that guidelines for diagnosis and treatment of OSA vary widely throughout the world. In many countries, OSA treatment will be done predominantly with CPAP, or to a lesser extend with MADs with only a limited role for UA surgery. DISE is also not reimbursed in many countries. Such local financial limitations restrict the widespread use of DISE.

While many sleep surgery experts advocate that DISE should be performed in all patients who will undergo UA surgery, others perform DISE only "on indication." It is the opinion of the authors of this book that DISE should always be performed in case sleep surgery is considered, unless there are good reasons not to do it.

5.3 DISE in Naive OSA Patients

The most obvious indication for DISE is a naive OSA patient who seeks help for treatment of his/her OSA. The patient wants to know his/her options and wants to take a decision to go for a certain therapy only after all information is available and all pros and cons of all different treatment modalities have been weighed. The decision to commence with a certain treatment might have lifelong consequences. After the sleep study, when the diagnosis OSA is confirmed, a global discussion about potential different treatment options follows. While the patient understands that CPAP is an option, he/she still want to be informed about possible alternatives before embarking on lifelong CPAP treatment.

In such a case, when all treatment modalities are still open, DISE is performed. Already the same day that DISE takes place, or later, the DISE observations can be discussed with the patient, and based on the results of the combined sleep study and DISE findings, the advantages and disadvantages of all conservative, surgical, and non-surgical treatment modalities are discussed. In addition to CPAP, the pro and cons of MAD are discussed: based on the DISE and effect of maneuvers such as jaw thrust, or simulation bite, MAD treatment might be considered a good or bad idea. Sometimes the effect of jaw thrust in supine position is not good, but a better opening of the UA is observed in lateral position. This might be a consideration to add positional therapy to MAD treatment.[4]

5.4 DISE in Positional OSA

Another situation occurs in case a patient appears to be very positional after the sleep study: the number of events is much higher in supine position as compared to lateral sleep position. Should such a patient still have a DISE, or should positional therapy be offered first? If DISE is still performed in such a case, and if there is a great effect of turning from supine to lateral position alone already, this might be a reason to consider positional therapy as the only treatment to begin with, in particular since this finding is a confirmation of the large positional effect as earlier found in the polysomnography (PSG).

5.5 DISE and UA Surgery

Patients who do not want to be dependent on a device—be it CPAP, MAD, or positional device—can be informed about the site(s), configuration and severity of their obstructions, and how that would translate to surgical intervention(s). In case of surgery, patients can subsequently be informed about which procedure(s), expected outcome, success rate, complications, and morbidity. In this era of shared decision-making, this is the desired workup.

5.6 DISE in Simple Snorers

The standard workup of patients with loud socially disturbing snoring and suspicion of OSA includes a sleep study. In case the AHI is below 5 per hour, the diagnosis OSA is not confirmed and such a patient will have the diagnosis "simple snorer," "socially unacceptable snorer," "habitual snorer," or "nonapneic snorer." After discussion of lifestyle interventions (weight loss, abstinence of alcohol if applicable, ear plugs for the bed partner, sleeping apart, etc.), the three interventions it usually it boils down to are positional therapy,[5,6,7,8] MAD treatment, or surgery. All three options need to be discussed.

The patient and bed partner will usually be able to tell if there is an important difference in the loudness of the snoring between supine and nonsupine sleep position. A significant percentage (70%) of snorers are positional; their snore index is at least twice as high in supine sleeping position as compared to the other sleeping positions.[9] Usually, the sleep study will add information or confirm these differences as well. In case the snoring is mostly a supine sleep position issue, positional therapy could be offered first (if the new generation positional therapy devices are available).

Oral device therapy for snoring is successful in roughly 2/3 of cases.[10] The advice is usually to use a good—expensive—device; "one gets what one pays for" and it is very disappointing for a patient and his/her bed partner if the patient is the one out of three in whom MAD therapy is not successful. For this reason, it can be considered to perform DISE first before embarking on MAD treatment, even in simple snorers. It also depends on the local financial regulations. In the Netherlands, DISE is reimbursed even in simple snoring. In many other countries, it is not.

Regarding upper airway surgery for snoring, DISE is recommended or at least should be discussed with the patient and bed partner.

5.7 DISE after UA Surgery, MAD, and UA Stimulation Treatment Failure

Both after UA surgery, treatment with MAD, and UA stimulation, failures will occur in a certain percentage of the patients. In these situations, it is to be recommended to repeat DISE and perform a careful assessment of the reason of failure. In case of surgical failure, it is of utmost importance to assess the residual level of obstruction. Is it still the level(s) that were addressed with the surgery and/or has the obstruction pattern changed and how does this translate to additional treatment options, be it surgical or nonsurgical?

In case of MAD treatment failure, patients should be asked to bring their MAD and perform DISE both with and without MAD *in situ*.

In case of UAS failure, DISE with stimulation on and off in different modes and power settings can be very illuminating.[11] Not only is it helpful to find and fine-tune the optimal stimulation setting, it can also provide information on the stimulation effect on the different levels of obstruction. In many cases, UAS does not only open obstructions at the level of the tongue base but also at the level of the palate. This phenomenon is known as "coupling." In other cases, the effect on the tongue base is good, while there is little or no effect on palatal level. This might be reason to offer additional palatal surgery. In addition, other types of combination therapy might be thought of after revealing the results of the DISE in these cases.

5.8 DISE after Weight Loss

Improvement of severe OSA after weight loss to less severe pathology might be a reason to repeat DISE. This might be conducted either after dieting and exercise or after surgical weight loss. In case the DISE findings were unfavorable for surgery before weight loss (e.g., complete concentric palatal collapse and total obstruction at all other levels), the collapse pattern and severity might improve, and a patient might become a better candidate for UA surgery or UAS or MAD treatment, or might need less aggressive surgical intervention than would have been advised originally, before weight loss. After weight loss, improvement from CCCp to anteroposterior collapse has been observed on many occasions.

5.9 DISE and CPAP Failure

In spite of all improvements in CPAP devices provided by the CPAP industry, CPAP failure still happens in roughly 35% of patients.[12] There are many reasons for failure such as simple reluctance to use the machine, skin irritation, blocked nose, claustrophobia, mask leakage, and inability to fall asleep with it. In some cases, the reason for failure is unclear; the patient has no issue with the CPAP therapy but does not have the desired effect. In such a case, it can be considered to perform DISE with CPAP on. A small opening has to be made in the mask, large enough to pass the endoscope but not too big in order to avoid leakage. The reason for failure can in this way be assessed. In most, but not all, cases an epiglottic obstruction can be observed.[13]

References

[1] Vanderveken OM, Maurer JT, Hohenhorst W, et al. Evaluation of drug-induced sleep endoscopy as a patient selection tool for implanted upper airway stimulation for obstructive sleep apnea. J Clin Sleep Med. 2013; 9(5):433–438

[2] Strollo PJ, Jr, Soose RJ, Maurer JT, et al. STAR Trial Group. Upper-airway stimulation for obstructive sleep apnea. N Engl J Med. 2014; 370(2):139–149

[3] Op de Beeck S, Dieltjens M, Verbruggen AE, et al. Phenotypic labelling using drug-induced sleep endoscopy improves patient selection for mandibular advancement device outcome: a prospective study. J Clin Sleep Med. 2019; 15(8):1089–1099 Epub ahead of print

[4] Dieltjens M, Vroegop AV, Verbruggen AE, et al. A promising concept of combination therapy for positional obstructive sleep apnea. Sleep Breath. 2015; 19(2):637–644

[5] Ravesloot MJL, van Maanen JP, Dun L, de Vries N. The undervalued potential of positional therapy in position-dependent snoring and obstructive sleep apnea-a review of the literature. Sleep Breath. 2013; 17(1):39–49

[6] van Maanen JP, Richard W, Van Kesteren ER, et al. Evaluation of a new simple treatment for positional sleep apnoea patients. J Sleep Res. 2012; 21(3):322–329

[7] van Maanen JP, de Vries N. Long-term effectiveness and compliance of positional therapy with the sleep position trainer in the treatment of positional obstructive sleep apnea syndrome. Sleep (Basel). 2014; 37(7):1209–1215

[8] Benoist L, de Ruiter M, de Lange J, de Vries N. A randomized, controlled trial of positional therapy versus oral appliance therapy for position-dependent sleep apnea. Sleep Med. 2017; 34:109–117

[9] Benoist LBL, Morong S, van Maanen JP, Hilgevoord AAJ, de Vries N. Evaluation of position dependency in non-apneic snorers. Eur Arch Otorhinolaryngol. 2014; 271(1):189–194

[10] Ferguson KA, Cartwright R, Rogers R, Schmidt-Nowara W. Oral appliances for snoring and obstructive sleep apnea: a review. Sleep. 2006; 29(2):244–262

[11] Safiruddin F, Vanderveken OM, de Vries N, et al. Effect of upper-airway stimulation for obstructive sleep apnoea on airway dimensions. Eur Respir J. 2015; 45(1):129–138

[12] Richard W, Venker J, den Herder C, et al. Acceptance and long-term compliance of nCPAP in obstructive sleep apnea. Eur Arch Otorhinolaryngol. 2007; 264(9):1081–1086

[13] Dedhia RC, Rosen CA, Soose RJ. What is the role of the larynx in adult obstructive sleep apnea? Laryngoscope. 2014; 124(4):1029–1034

6 Preparation for DISE: Informed Consent

Marc Blumen

Abstract

An example of an informed consent form is provided, as used in Hôpital Foch, Paris, France. This can serve as a template and might also be modified according to local circumstances.

Keywords: obstructive sleep apnea, drug-induced sleep endoscopy, informed consent

6.1 Introduction

In drug-induced sleep endoscopy (DISE), as in all procedures, patient information is mandatory. Below is an example of an informed consent form, as used in Hôpital Foch, Paris, France. It can serve as an example and might also be modified according to local circumstances.

Dear Patient,

You are about to undergo DISE, which is a diagnostic examination consisting of putting you to sleep and visualizing the site or sites of vibration and obstruction responsible for your snoring and, if present, sleep apnea.

This examination will enable the doctor and yourself to choose the best suited treatment in your specific case. The earlier sleep study was conducted to be informed about the severity of your disease; DISE is helpful in obtaining a better understanding of the cause of your problem.

DISE is performed in an ambulatory setting. Once the examination is carried out, you will need to stay in the recovery room or ward for several hours until you are fully awake. It is recommended that somebody picks you up and takes you home.

DISE is performed in an operating room or special endoscopy suite. An intravenous line will be put in place and electrodes placed on your chest to monitor your heart rate; a cuff will be positioned around your arm to monitor your blood pressure and a clip on one of your fingers to monitor your blood oxygen saturation.

An anesthesiologist or specialized nurse will inject a sedative drug intravenously to help you fall asleep. You will breath by yourself. Sometimes, the deepness of your sleep will be monitored by placing a band on your forehead.

Once you are asleep, the doctor will pass a flexible endoscope through the left or right side of your nose, depending on which side is the widest. Extra medication might be needed to make the examination easier, such as atropine to decrease the amount of saliva, or local anesthetics and/or nose drops to reduce swelling of the nasal mucosa, in order to avoid waking you up during the examination.

Once asleep and down several levels of depth of sedation, the doctor will evaluate the different sites of obstruction and vibration at the level of the soft palate, side walls of the throats, tonsils (when still present), tongue, and epiglottis (larynx). The images of your throat will be viewed on a screen and may be recorded. Maneuvers which simulate different situations will be performed during the DISE, such as pulling the lower jaw forward to mimic what an oral appliance could do for you, put you on the side, or turn your head sideways to mimic positional therapy and observe which obstruction and vibration sites remain.

Putting a silicone tube down the nasal cavity in your throat could also be part of the examination, in order to test the validity of the obstruction sites seen, particularly at the level of the tongue base and the epiglottis. The tube length needed to pass the soft palate, or the obstruction lower down in the throat, may be measured.

The examination lasts between 15 and 40 minutes, depending on how fast you fall asleep and the occurrence of the obstruction/vibration sites.

No serious side effects have ever been observed. Decrease in oxygen saturation induced by the examination can occur. This is actually what happens every night during your sleep hours. The anesthesiologist will be cautious not to let the oxygen saturation go lower than what happens in your natural sleep. It is almost never necessary to give oxygen or use a continuous positive airway pressure (CPAP) machine with a mask placed on the nose and face. Placement of a tube for breathing is hardly ever needed and extremely rare. Excess salivation can make optimal assessment of the airway difficult. In order to have as good as possible view of the inside of your throat, it might be necessary to suck saliva away during examination. Aspiration of saliva is extremely rare.

The passage of the fibroscope through the nasal cavity can induce sneezing and excess secretions, and make visualization more difficult. A little bleeding of the nasal mucosa might occur but is usually self-limiting. Finally, in rare cases, snoring cannot be reliably reproduced and therefore DISE will not be helpful in orientation toward a specific therapy for your snoring and apnea.

---

7 Organization and Logistics

Linda Benoist and Nico de Vries

Abstract

In this chapter, we share our experience—in a how-we-do-it fashion—about drug-induced sleep endoscopy (DISE) as standard diagnostic tool for patients with obstructive sleep apnea (OSA), where non-continuous positive airway pressure (CPAP) therapies are considered. In case of a large numbers of such patients, efficient organization of the procedure and logistics become critically important. In our experience, DISE can be performed by an ENT resident and nurse anesthetist in an outpatient endoscopy setting without issues in patients with American Society of Anesthesiologists (ASA) I or II. The use of a standardized DISE scoring system such as the velum, oropharynx, tongue base, and epiglottis (VOTE) score allows a common framework for reporting DISE findings.

Keywords: sleep apnea, drug-induced sleep endoscopy, logistics, organization

7.1 Introduction

Drug-induced sleep endoscopy (DISE) has gradually changed from an experimental diagnostic modality to an established form of upper airway (UA) assessment in patients receiving non-continuous positive airway pressure (CPAP) therapies for sleep-disordered breathing (SDB). Clinical and scientific interest in DISE is rapidly growing.[1]

The growing number of DISEs has consequences for the organization of clinical protocols and DISE research. When DISE is performed occasionally, it can be incorporated in a regular operation room (OR) schedule. However, if many DISEs are performed routinely on a weekly basis, other more efficient forms of organizations might be preferable.

With ever increasing numbers of DISEs, several organizational and logistical questions should be considered:

- Does DISE need to be performed by the same surgeon who would perform the sleep surgery, or can it be also carried out by another staff member or even a medical resident without the presence of a senior staff member?
- Is it necessary to perform DISE in the OR, or can it be conducted safely in an outpatient setting?
- Is the presence of an anesthesiologist necessary or can sedation be provided by a nurse anesthetist?
- Is it necessary that the endoscopist (or person who performs the DISE) discusses the DISE findings with the patient after the procedure, or can someone else from the care team do this?
- Can the post-DISE consultation be done on the same day or should the patient and bed partner come back for a separate consultation?

In this how-we-do-it chapter, we share our recent experiences. In otherwise healthy patients, DISE is performed by an ENT resident, with sedation provided by a dedicated nurse anesthetist, in an outpatient endoscopy setting, while the staff member/sleep surgeon discusses the findings and the recommended treatment proposal often on the same day.

7.2 Materials and Methods

7.2.1 History of DISE in Our Hospital

The department of Otolaryngology at the OLVG West Hospital in Amsterdam, The Netherlands, serves as a referral center for treating patients with SDB. Since 20 years, DISE has been performed. Presently, approximately 3000 sleep studies, the majority being full night polysomnography's (PSGs), more than 800 DISE's, and around 200 sleep surgeries (excluding nasal surgery) are performed on an annual basis. While DISE was originally performed in case UA surgery was considered, we now also perform DISE in case upper airway stimulation (UAS, Chapter 18 and Chapter 20), positional therapy (Chapter 11), mandibular advancement device (MAD) therapy (Chapter 22), or combined treatments are considered.

7.2.2 Patient Indication for DISE

Our selection criteria for DISE are as follows: mild to moderate obstructive sleep apnea (OSA) (i.e., apnea–hypopnea index [AHI] between 5 and 30/h sleep), severe OSA and CPAP failure, body mass index (BMI) <32/ kg/m², potential candidates for UA surgery, UAS, oral appliance therapy (OAT) and positional therapy (PT) or combination treatment in specific cases, and American Society of Anesthesiologists (ASA) I or II. ASA 3 and severe cardiovascular comorbidity are relative contraindications for the outpatient endoscopy setting, and these patients still have their DISE performed in the OR. Selecting lower BMI is important, as it has been shown that surgery and oral devices have lower success rates above this BMI threshold.[2,3,4] There are exceptions to this rule: patients with relatively much abdominal fat and normal neck circumference might still be good candidates for UA surgery or UAS.

7.2.3 Staff

Already in January 2013, we switched from having an ENT staff performing DISE in the OR to performing the DISE in an outpatient endoscopy setting. The DISE is performed by an ENT resident, with a trained nurse anesthetist managing sedation. The other personnel present in the room is the ENT doctors' assistant, who arranges the flexible nasal endoscope, presets the video recording system, and assists with minimizing patient movement during the examination. After DISE, patients go into a recovery area where a recovery nurse monitors blood pressure and saturation levels and gives oxygen as needed.

7.2.4 Sedation Protocol

In the outpatient endoscopy setting, we monitor blood pressure, pulse oximetry, and electrocardiogram (ECG) during DISE. To preoxygenate the patient, 100% oxygen by face mask is given. While in the past midazolam sedation was used, we have stopped doing this, mainly because of the amnesia caused by midazolam, which excludes the possibility to discuss the DISE outcome with the patient on the same day. Currently, we use intravenous propofol with the sedation rate controlled by a target-controlled infusion (TCI) pump.

The sedation starts by setting the TCI pump according to height, age, and body weight of the patient. Prior to the propofol, we administer 2 mL lidocaine through the IV to prevent pain caused by the infusion of propofol. In case indicated, glycopyrrolate (antisecretory drug) will be given intravenously to avoid excessive secretions, which may interfere with the quality of the imaging. The initial sedation starts with a small bolus of propofol (20–50 mg) and then maintained by the TCI pump. When the patient does not respond to the eyelash reflex and questions and/or starts snoring, the nasal endoscope is introduced. Adverse effects of the DISE procedure are rare; we have never encountered severe side effects or emergency situations.

7.2.5 Logistics

Once the patient is approved for DISE during the preprocedure review, the OR planner will schedule the patient. In our outpatient endoscopy setting, we have six beds available, and patients undergo DISE in series, meaning one patient comes in for DISE as the last patient goes back out to postanesthesia recovery.

As a rule, all patients will have at least four assessments: one in supine position, one in supine position with jaw thrust, one in lateral position, and one in lateral position with jaw thrust. On indication, even more assessments are performed, for example, patients who experienced MAD treatment failure might undergo DISE with their MAD in situ as well, again in both positions. Sometimes turning of the head might provide almost the same information as rotation of both head and trunk (Chapter 11). In this way, it is possible to perform seven cases/half day session. Roughly half of the patients come from outside the Amsterdam region; they will be offered a same day consultation with the sleep surgeon to discuss the results and treatment options.

7.2.6 DISE Report

After the DISE, the ENT resident composes a report which includes the following:

- Results of the previous PSG containing, at a minimum, the AHI (obstructive, mixed, and central), and the AHI's in each sleeping position. As a rule all patients will have a PSG first and only after that will DISE be performed.
- BMI and ENT investigation findings, including nasal examination and dental status.
- The velum, oropharynx, tongue base, and epiglottis (VOTE) score is used to classify the UA collapse pattern during DISE, which is also video recorded for later review if needed.[5,6] In case an oral device is considered as treatment option, a jaw thrust is performed. Similarly, if positional therapy may be considered, the DISE will also be performed with the patient's head in a lateral position.[7,8,9,10,11]
- The resident's treatment proposal might include the following: conservative measures, CPAP, oral device, positional therapy, various forms of UA surgery and UAS, participation in clinical trials, or combined therapies.[12,13,14] This report allows the supervisor to check the resident's progress with regard to their train of thought at diagnosis and treatment of patient.

7.3 Results

The results presented here were published earlier elsewhere. Between April 2012 and September 2014, in total ±950 DISE's (2012: ±120, 2013: ±480, and 2014: ±350) were performed by an ENT resident and nurse anesthetist in an outpatient endoscopy setting. On average, the typical DISE lasts 15 minutes. No complications or fatalities have ever occurred in this period or in the approximately 20 years before. After DISE, patients spend on average 60 to 90 minutes in the recovery room, and are then sufficiently awake to attend an office consultation to discuss the DISE findings and therapeutic options.

7.4 Discussion

The department of otolaryngology at the OLVG West Hospital in Amsterdam, The Netherlands, serves as a referral center for treating patients with SDB. A considerable number of patients visit the outward clinic because they want to be informed about possible alternatives to CPAP. The Dutch guideline for diagnosis and treatment of OSA in adults leaves room for all types of treatment: CPAP, OAT, positional therapy, UA surgery and UAS, and bariatric surgery. In The Netherlands, DISE as a diagnostic tool for assessment of the UA is widely accepted.

DISE is a standard diagnostic tool for patients with OSA in our hospital where non-CPAP therapies are considered. Because of the large numbers of such patients in our clinic, organization of procedure logistics becomes critically important. One day a week, in otherwise healthy patients (ASA I and II), 14 DISE procedures are performed, seven in the morning and seven in the afternoon in a day care endoscopy setting, by an ENT resident and dedicated anesthetist nurse practitioner. In addition, patients with ASA III or IV will have their DISE in the operating theatre with an anesthetist present.

The use of a standardized DISE scoring system such as the VOTE score allows a common framework for sharing findings between the endoscopist (who now as a routine is an ENT resident) and the ENT surgeon. In some cases, further discussion of the DISE findings between the resident and staff surgeon might be indicated, for example, in case of complete circular palatal collapse versus anteroposterior collapse, as this might have consequences for eligibility of certain forms of surgery such as UAS. In these circumstances, the DISE video recordings can be reassessed by the resident, surgeon, or a larger group in order to reach consensus. From a teaching perspective, there is also an advantage of delegating DISE to the resident. This system allows the supervisor to monitor the resident's logic and learning while performing a large number of DISE procedures, as it has been well-established that high-procedure volume is important for proper medical training.

7.5 Conclusion

In our experience, DISE can be safely performed in an outpatient endoscopy setting by an ENT resident and nurse anesthetist. This system is safe, efficient, and improves patient access to care by combining the DISE with post-DISE evaluation on the same day.

Acknowledgment

The authors would like to thank the following nurse anesthetists for their help and valuable support during the DISE procedures: P. Karlas, E. van Aalst, and A. van Limburg-Brouwer.

References

[1] De Vito A, Carrasco Llatas M, Vanni A, et al. European position paper on drug-induced sedation endoscopy (DISE). Sleep Breath. 2014; 18 (3):453–465

[2] Gislason T, Lindholm CE, Almqvist M, et al. Uvulopalatopharyngoplasty in the sleep apnea syndrome. Predictors of results. Arch Otolaryngol Head Neck Surg. 1988; 114(1):45–51

[3] Kezirian EJ, Goldberg AN. Hypopharyngeal surgery in obstructive sleep apnea: an evidence-based medicine review. Arch Otolaryngol Head Neck Surg. 2006; 132(2):206–213

[4] Kezirian EJ, Malhotra A, Goldberg AN, White DP. Changes in obstructive sleep apnea severity, biomarkers, and quality of life after multilevel surgery. Laryngoscope. 2010; 120(7):1481–1488

[5] Kezirian EJ, Hohenhorst W, de Vries N. Drug-induced sleep endoscopy: the VOTE classification. Eur Arch Otorhinolaryngol. 2011; 268(8): 1233–1236

[6] Ravesloot MJL, de Vries N. One hundred consecutive patients undergoing drug-induced sleep endoscopy: results and evaluation. Laryngoscope. 2011; 121(12):2710–2716

[7] Ravesloot MJ, van Maanen JP, Dun L, de Vries N. The undervalued potential of positional therapy in position-dependent snoring and obstructive sleep apnea-a review of the literature. Sleep Breath. 2013; 17(1):39–49

[8] van Maanen JP, Meester KA, Dun LN, et al. The sleep position trainer: a new treatment for positional obstructive sleep apnoea. Sleep Breath. 2013; 17(2):771–779

[9] van Maanen JP, Richard W, Van Kesteren ER, et al. Evaluation of a new simple treatment for positional sleep apnoea patients. J Sleep Res. 2012; 21(3):322–329

[10] Safiruddin F, Koutsourelakis I, de Vries N. Analysis of the influence of head rotation during drug-induced sleep endoscopy in obstructive sleep apnea. Laryngoscope. 2014; 124(9):2195–2199

[11] Safiruddin F, Koutsourelakis I, de Vries N. Upper airway collapse during drug-induced sleep endoscopy: head rotation in supine position compared with lateral head and trunk position. Eur Arch Otorhinolaryngol. 2014

[12] Strollo PJ, Jr, Soose RJ, Maurer JT, et al. STAR Trial Group. Upper-airway stimulation for obstructive sleep apnea. N Engl J Med. 2014; 370(2):139–149

[13] Vanderveken OM, Maurer JT, Hohenhorst W, et al. Evaluation of drug-induced sleep endoscopy as a patient selection tool for implanted upper airway stimulation for obstructive sleep apnea. J Clin Sleep Med. 2013; 9(5):433–438

[14] Vroegop AV, Vanderveken OM, Boudewyns AN, et al. Drug-induced sleep endoscopy in sleep-disordered breathing: report on 1,249 cases. Laryngoscope. 2014; 124(3):797–802

8 Patient Preparation and Positioning

Srinivas Kishore S.

Abstract

In this chapter, an overview is provided of preoperative evaluation, operation theatre preparation, patient preparation, patient positioning, endoscopist positioning, and interventional drug-induced sleep endoscopy (DISE).

Keywords: drug-induced sleep endoscopy, preparation, positioning

8.1 Introduction

Obstructive sleep apnea (OSA) is sleep-associated respiratory distress characterized by snoring, and it could be a complete or incomplete airway obstruction that repeatedly occurs during sleep, which leads to decreased blood oxygen saturation. Patients with OSA show anatomical abnormalities of the upper airways and physiological alterations.

Continuous positive airway pressure (CPAP) devices or oral appliances may be used for OSA treatment. Surgical treatments including maxillomandibular advancement (MMA) may also be performed. Drug-induced sleep endoscopy (DISE) is a method to visually identify the causes of upper airway obstruction to increase the success rate of OSA treatment. Drug-induced sleep induction must be performed to induce snoring before performing DISE. Anesthetics such as propofol, midazolam, and dexmedetomidine are primarily used for this procedure. To increase the DISE success rate, drugs that induce near-normal sleep should be administered, and sleep and snoring must be maintained by ensuring anesthetics are within appropriate concentration ranges. However, when deep sedation is induced in a patient with OSA until the patient begins to snore, airway obstruction may become more severe than expected, and the patient may stop breathing, resulting in decreased oxygen saturation. Airway management must be performed, and airway interventions such as cardiopulmonary resuscitation (CPR) may be necessary. Oxygen administration is essential in DISE, and clinicians must monitor patients carefully to ensure respiratory failure or airway obstruction does not occur.

8.2 Preoperative Preparation

The most important task for the surgeon is communication with the patient, and he or she has to discuss the goals of the OSA surgery with the patient. He has to explain the purpose of this DISE. Will the proposed OSA surgery be for cure or for palliation?

Once the patient understands the importance of this procedure, then the surgeon needs to communicate the idea of DISE, how it will be done, and what are the possible complications of this procedure?

Most importantly, the surgeon needs to discuss with the anaesthesia team. It is ideal to have a preferred anesthesiologist who understands the goal of DISE. Snoring that leads to witnessed OSA is the goal of DISE, and the anesthesiologist must not be afraid of obstructive events on the table. Desaturations are expected and should be tolerated within reason. It is helpful to point out that patients with OSA experience obstructive episodes and desaturations continually in the privacy of their own bedroom.

We can perform DISE immediately before the proposed OSA surgery. Any planned nasal surgery can be easily decided in the clinic, but the DISE findings can definitely influence which oropharyngeal and/or hypopharyngeal procedure is to be performed on the patient. So, we have to discuss every possible scenario with the patient during the counseling purposes.

Another alternative is to perform DISE in the operating room and then perform the definitive surgery after the sleep endoscopy discussion in the clinic. This is helpful when we do staged, multilevel surgery. We can perform DISE and nasal surgery and then bring the patient back for oropharyngeal/hypopharyngeal OSA surgery. Then, we have to discuss the findings of the DISE with the patient and decide upon the definitive procedure in the palate or/and tongue base.

8.3 Operation Theatre Preparation

The following equipment needed for the procedure needs to be kept ready:
- Audiovisual (AV) system: An AV system with recording capability is a great way to review cases and improve one's decision algorithm and technique; the recordings also make great teaching tools for staff, patients, residents, and students.
- A microphone is optional to record airway sounds and snoring.
- Adjustable operating table.
- Monitors for pulse oximetry and routine vital signs.
- Oxygen and mask and/or nasal cannula; air mask bag unit (AMBU).
- Target-controlled infusion (TCI) pump.
- Bispectral index (BIS) monitor.
- Flexible laryngoscope with defogging solution of choice.
- Flexible suction and Yankauer suction.

By definition, patients with OSA have potentially difficult airways. While it is rare to lose an airway by this method, one must always be prepared for the worst case scenario. Equipment for intubation of emergent airways should be ready and it includes the following:

- Tracheotomy tray.
- Laryngoscope with various Miller and Macintosh blades.
- Magill forceps.
- Laryngeal mask airways (LMAs) and intubating LMAs.
- Eschmann stylet.
- Combitube.
- Endotracheal tubes of various sizes.
- Jet ventilation and 14-gauge needle.
- Nasopharyngeal airway.
- Oropharyngeal airway.

8.4 Patient Preparation

Complete hemogram, lipid profile, liver, kidney and thyroid function tests, chest radiograph, and ECG need to be done.

After getting the informed written consent, the patient will be kept nil oral for 6 hours.

Medications administered to the patient include the following:

Single IV dose of glycopyrrolate 0.2 mg can be administered in the preoperative suite at least 15 minutes prior to DISE; it will decrease the salivary secretions, allowing optimal viewing during DISE.

Oxymetazoline nasal spray: Two sprays into both nostrils 15 minutes prior to the procedure will be ideal.

It is better to avoid any topical lidocaine, as this could potentially remove and blunt any natural airway reflexes. At the same time, to reduce nasal and intraoral stimulation during nasoendoscopy, local anesthesia can be administered as a 2% Lidocaine gel in both sides of the nasal cavity.

Patient will be taken into the operation room without premedication.

A noninvasive blood pressure monitor, pulse oximetry, ECG, and BIS sensor will be attached. Before inducing the patient, oxygen saturation, blood pressure, and breathing rate will be measured and recorded.

To encourage sleep, lights to be dimmed and noise should be minimized. A total of 3 mL of 1% Lidocaine will be intravenously administered for pain reduction within blood vessels, when propofol will be intravenously injected using a syringe pump system through TCI to induce sedation.

8.5 Patient Positioning

Positioning of the patient plays a pivotal role while performing DISE. Patients by habit sleep in different positions such as supine, lateral and prone. The most ideal way to perform will be in the position that the patient adopts during his or her natural daily sleep. This information gathered from polysomnography (PSG) can be utilized in positioning the patient for DISE, especially for a patient with positional OSA. Since the procedure involves turning the patient, it is suggested that the bed is wide enough for the staff to help in maneuvering the sedated patient during the procedure.

Routinely, DISE is performed with the patient in supine position; it can also be performed with head tilt or head and trunk toward the lateral positions. Various studies suggest that DISE findings differ when performed in different positions.[1] However, studies by Safiruddin et al have shown that the findings remain the same when performed with just the head rotation or head and neck rotation.[2] This topic is fully covered in Chapter 11.

8.6 Positioning of the Endoscopist in Performing DISE

The procedure can be performed either by standing at the head end of the patient or beside the patient.

Some patients with OSA are habitual mouth breathers and hence in order to assess their upper airway during sleep, it is advisable to perform transoral DISE. Transoral DISE will not only highlight the severity of tongue base collapse secondary to impaired tone but may also be secondary to a tongue base collapse, if the finding is suggestive of an AP collapse at the palate on nasopharyngoscopy; hence, the pattern can be falsely reported.

Types of scope entry:
- Transnasal.
- Transoral.

8.7 Interventional DISE

OSA is a condition caused by obstructions at multiple levels, among which palatal level is the commonest.[4] Interventional DISE is a more dynamic approach wherein the endoscopist actively manipulates the upper airway with either a nasopharyngeal airway or a MAD.[5] This intervention which mimics different treatment modalities helps the endoscopist to change the behavior of the upper airway accordingly to prognosticate outcomes.

- Nasopharyngeal airway: The placement of nasopharyngeal airway is one of the tools in the treatment armamentarium of OSA. Li et al demonstrated that nasopharyngeal tube placement and PSG identified patients who would benefit from uvulopalatopharyngoplasty (UPPP) alone as opposed to a multilevel surgery.[6] It has also been shown that nasopharyngeal airway helps mimic the impact of palatal surgery on the airway. The benefit of this has been observed maximum on the lateral wall and epiglottis collapse. However, the benefit could not be extended to tongue base collapse.

- Mandibular advancing device: MAD prevents upper airway collapse by protruding the mandible forward, thus altering the jaw and tongue position. This helps relieve obstruction not only at level of the tongue base but also at the level of the velum, due to traction on soft-tissue connections between the pharynx and the mandibular ramus.[7] However, this treatment modality cannot applied to every patient.

While performing DISE, it is recommended to perform the ESMARCH maneuver, which involves pulling the mandible upward and forward with the head slightly extended to retract the tongue from the posterior pharyngeal wall.[8] This procedure helps to prognosticate the efficacy of MAD as a treatment modality. There is evidence that a hyper-protrusion/maximal protrusion of the mandible has no predictive value toward the opioid against treatment (OAT) outcome. Therefore, performing a maximal mandibular protrusion maneuver is not advisable. If the patient's own device is available, it is recommended that the DISE be performed with the device in situ before starting the sedation.[9] When available, the use of a simulation bite in maximal comfortable protrusion (MCP) of the mandible during DISE is recommended in patients with OSA, which could be effective in predicting treatment response of MAD.[9] The topic is further covered in Chapter 11.

8.8 Conclusion

The safest way to perform sleep endoscopy involves a team approach with your anesthesiologist, and DISE performed in a monitored setting. As described above, communication with your patient and the operative team is important.

In order to get a reliable and valid examination, patience is needed. Allow the chosen drug to work and allow the patient to settle down into snoring and then an eventual obstruction; thereafter, record the findings.

References

[1] Lee CH, Kim DK, Kim SY, Rhee CS, Won TB. Changes in site of obstruction in obstructive sleep apnea patients according to sleep position: a DISE study. Laryngoscope. 2015; 125(1):248–254

[2] Safiruddin F, Koutsourelakis I, de Vries N. Upper airway collapse during drug induced sleep endoscopy: head rotation in supine position compared with lateral head and trunk position. Eur Arch Otorhinolaryngol. 2015; 272(2):485–488

[3] Ravesloot MJ, de Vries N. One hundred consecutive patients undergoing drug-induced sleep endoscopy: results and evaluation. Laryngoscope. 2011; 121(12):2710–2716

[4] Victores AJ, Olson, K, Takashima, M. Interventional drug-induced sleep endoscopy: a novel technique to guide surgical planning for obstructive sleep apnea. J Clinic Sleep Med. 2017; 13(2): 169–174

[5] Li S, Wu D, Bao J, Qin J. Nasopharyngeal tube: a simple and effective tool to screen patients indicated for glossopharyngeal surgery. J Clin Sleep Med. 2014; 10(4):385–389

[6] Brown EC, Cheng S, McKenzie DK, Butler JE, Gandevia SC, Bilston LE. Respiratory movement of upper airway tissue in obstructive sleep apnea. Sleep (Basel). 2013; 36(7):1069–1076

[7] Kappeler O. Anaesthetica. Stuttgart: F. Enke; 1880

[8] De Vito A, Carrasco Llatas M, Ravesloot MJL, et al. European position paper on drug-induced sleep endoscopy: 2017 update. Clin Otolaryngol. 2018; 43(6):1541–1552

[9] Vroegop AVMT, Vanderveken OM, Van de Heyning PH, Braem MJ. Effects of vertical opening on pharyngeal dimensions in patients with obstructive sleep apnoea. Sleep Med. 2012; 13(3):314–316

9 Drugs for DISE

Evert Hamans and Marina Carrasco Llatas

Abstract

Obstructive sleep apnea (OSA) is a sleep-related breathing disorder where a partial or complete collapse of the upper airway (UA) results in nocturnal oxygen desaturation and poor-sleep quality. Drug-induced sleep endoscopy (DISE) has become a widespread diagnostic tool to localize and quantify different collapse patterns that guides the physician to a tailor-made therapeutic approach for these patients. In order to mimic natural sleep, the choice of drug used and its administration is crucial in order to make DISE a reliable, safe, and representable way of phenotyping UA collapse in OSA patients.

Keywords: obstructive sleep apnea, airway management, sedation, natural sleep, drug-induced sleep

9.1 Introduction

Drug-induced sleep endoscopy (DISE) is a diagnostic tool for patients with obstructive sleep apnea (OSA). It is an endoscopic observation of the level(s), degree and pattern of obstruction of the upper airway (UA) during drug-induced sleep/sedation. UA evaluation in awake OSA patients has limited usefulness, since the level of collapse during sleep can be significantly different to those observed in awake patients, primarily due to differences in muscle tone during sleep. The scientific basis for the varied combinations of pharmacological agents and delivery algorithms is tenuous.[1] To choose an ideal agent, one must match the current understanding of sleep-related neurophysiology to that of sedation-induced neuropharmacology.

The neurophysiology of sleep breathing is quite complex. However, there are basic elements that must be understood. Obstruction during sleep occurs primarily during nonrapid eye movement (NREM)1/NREM2 and rapid eye movement (REM) sleep, whereas NREM3 (delta sleep) is relatively obstruction-resistant.[2] Acetylcholine and gamma-aminobutyric acid (GABA) are the primary neurotransmitters for REM and NREM sleep, respectively. From this basic understanding of sleep neurophysiology, the optimal DISE agent must possess certain characteristics (▶ Table 9.1).[3] In practice, onset of action, medication half-life, and amnestic properties are of clinical importance. In order to mimic natural sleep, it is crucial that drug-induced sleep is created with the use of drug(s) that mimic natural sleep as optimal as possible, mimic the collapsibility of the UA as optimal as possible, all within feasibility and safety limits.

Table 9.1 Neurophysiologic characteristics for ideal agents for DISE

Reproduction of:
- Stage NREM1, NREM2, and/or REM sleep

Preservation of:
- Mechanoreceptor input to brainstem
- Chemoreceptor input to brainstem
- Respiratory rhythmicity by pre-Botzinger complex
- Lower cranial nerve motor output to pharyngolarynx

Abbreviations: NREM, nonrapid eye movement; REM, rapid eye movement.

9.2 Effects of Local Anesthesia and Nasal Decongestion

In the literature, nasal decongestion, nasal local anesthesia, and antisecretory drugs are described as preparatory measures and may be used as an option. Local anesthetics may be used during DISE in order to introduce the endoscope without sneezing. These agents scan potentially interact with UA and breathing control and have to be used with caution. The use of atropine-like agents in patients with excessive secretions may influence sleep physiology and is therefore not recommended. The use of local anesthesia or decongestants may increase the ease of scope insertion and possibly reduce the incidence of nasal irritation. These drugs could interfere with nasal resistance and, consequently, airflow.[4]

9.3 Drugs Used for DISE

There is a great variability in the drug or combination of drugs used for DISE reported in the literature. Basically, midazolam and propofol are the two drugs most widely used.[3]

Both propofol and midazolam are suitable as sedative agents, alone or in combination, with advantages and disadvantages. Most of the evidence that compares natural sleep and sedation is performed with propofol or midazolam as a single agent for sedation. Therefore, these are the drugs that should be used for DISE, as they provide a state that mimics the critical closing pressure during natural sleep without significant differences in the apnea–hypopnea index (AHI).[5,6]

Great care should be taken to avoid an overdose of the sedative agent and limit excessive muscle relaxation, resulting in overrating the UA collapse as a consequence.

▶ Table 9.2 shows the advantages and disadvantages of propofol, midazolam, and their combination.

Table 9.2 Advantages and disadvantages for sedative agents used for DISE

Sedative agents	Advantages	Disadvantages
Propofol	• Quick, safe, manageable • Less muscle relaxation • Easier control of titration	Technique dependent (MCI or TCI)
Midazolam	• Longer and more stable examination window • Midazolam antidote available	• More difficult to handle in case of overdosing • Longer hospital stay
Combined (P + M)	• Quicker and more stable mimicking of natural sleep • Midazolam antidote available	• Technique dependent (MCI or TCI) • Increases sneezing

9.3.1 Propofol

The exact mechanism of action of propofol is unknown. It is a global central nervous system depressant that activate GABA-A receptors directly. Propofol induces anesthesia quickly and is metabolized quickly. High-density EEG data are used to examine the differences in the cortical processes between propofol sedation and natural sleep. It was found that the onset of sedation resulted in the presence of slow waves that were similar to those found in natural NREM sleep. Also, propofol-induced slow waves originated in areas similar to those of natural sleep and traveled along similar neural pathways. However, propofol slow waves do not induce sleep spindle activity, in contrast to natural sleep.[7]

Onset of action is 15 to 30 seconds, biological half-life is 30 to 60 minutes, and duration of action is 5 to 10 minutes.

9.3.2 Midazolam

Midazolam is a GABA receptor agonist that produces sedative–hypnotic, anxiolytic, anticonvulsant, and muscle-relaxant effects.[8] Midazolam has been shown to have depressant effects on central respiratory drive, causing a decrease in ventilatory response to CO_2.[9]

Critical closing pressure (Pcrit) is not significantly different during natural sleep and midazolam sedation. Pcrit values are highly associated with the AHI, as determined by polysomnography (PSG), during both natural sleep and midazolam sedation. Sleep architecture is found to be similar between natural sleep and midazolam sedation. Therefore, it seems that midazolam sedation does not affect pharyngeal muscle tonicity or sleep architecture.[10]

Onset of action is within 5 minutes, biological half-life is 1.5 to 2.5 hours, and duration of action is 1 to 6 hours. Flumazenil can be used as an antidote.

9.3.3 Dexmedetomidine

Dexmedetomidine is an α_2-adrenergic agonist that effects neurons throughout the brain to produce sedation, sympatolytic effects, and analgesia. Although the exact mechanism that produces sedation is unknown, studies have suggested that dexmedetomidine acts on the locus Ceruleus (LC) to decrease wakefulness. Sleep spindles are quantitatively and qualitatively comparable in natural sleep and dexmedetomidine sedation. Similar spindle-generating neuronal mechanisms are found in both normal physiological NREM stage 2 sleep and N3 dexmedetomidine sedation.[11]

Onset of action is 10 minutes and elimination half-life is 2 to 3 hours. Dexmedetomidine has to be used with caution in patients already at risk of arrythmias and unstable cardiac status, or currently using of β-blocker, calcium channel blocker or digoxin.

9.4 Dosage of Drugs

9.4.1 Dosage of Propofol

There are three ways in which propofol can be administered: with target-controlled infusion (TCI), standard pump, or manual bolus injection (► Table 9.3).

The use of a syringe infusion pump with TCI technology as the standard mode for sedation is recommended when propofol is used, as it provides a more stable and reliable sedation than manual infusion schemes or bolus technique.[12] If a TCI infusion pump is not available, then a syringe infusion pump for manually controlled infusion is better than bolus. Most of the patients achieve an adequate level of sedation at an effective site concentration of 3.2 µg/mL. Therefore, a starting dose of 3.0 µg/mL could be applied, instead of the more conservative dose of 2.0 to 2.5 µg/mL, in order to achieve a quicker sedation. However, the physician has to keep in mind that if the sedation is achieved too quickly, more central apneas can occur in the beginning, creating a false image of obstruction.[13]

TCI

Starting dose: 2.0 to 2.5 µg/mL (effective site concentration). As some patients will not fall asleep with this starting dose, an increasing dose of 0.2 to 0.3 µg/mL every 2 minutes is suggested until the patient begins to snore and vibration and collapse of the UA is observed.

Table 9.3 Drug dosages and administration for the different drugs used during DISE

Schedule	Drug dosage	
	Midazolam	Propofol
Propofol alone		TCI (effect site concentration): • Starting dose: 2.0–2.5 µg/mL • If required, increase dose of 0.2–0.5 µg/mL every 2 min Manually controlled infusion: • Delivering dose: 50–100 mL/h Bolus technique: • Propofol 1, starting dose: 30–50 mg, increasing rate of 10 mg every 2 min • Propofol 2, starting dose: 1 mg/kg, increasing rate of 30 mg every 2 min
Midazolam alone	Bolus technique: • Starting dose: 0.05 mg/kg • Observe 2–5 min • If required, increase dose of 0.015–0.03 mg/kg	
Midazolam and propofol	Midazolam single bolus before administration of propofol: • Single starting dose: 0.05 mg/kg	Propofol TCI (effect site concentration): • Starting dose: 1.5–3.0 µg/mL • If required, increase dose of 0.2–0.5 µg/mL

Manually Controlled Infusion

Delivering dose: 50 to 100 mL/h, depending on the patient response.

Bolus Technique

Starting dose: 30 to 50 mg, increasing rate of 10 mg every 2 minutes, or starting dose 1 mg/kg, increasing rate of 20 mg every 2 minutes.

9.4.2 Dosage of Midazolam

Bolus technique Starting dose: 0.05 mg/kg, observing 2 to 5 minutes, and increasing rate of 0.03 mg/kg only if patient is awake, then waiting for 5 minutes. If the patient is not completely asleep, further increase of rate is needed to 0.015 mg/kg.

Controlled infusion: no shared experiences or evidence in literature.

9.4.3 Dosage of Dexmedetomidine

Loading dose 1.5 mcg/kg in 10 minutes. When using a pump, 1 to 2 mcg/kg/h.

References

[1] Ehsan Z, Mahmoud M, Shott SR, Amin RS, Ishman SL. The effects of anesthesia and opioids on the upper airway: A systematic review. Laryngoscope. 2016; 126(1):270–284

[2] Ratnavadivel R, Chau N, Stadler D, Yeo A, McEvoy RD, Catcheside PG. Marked reduction in obstructive sleep apnea severity in slow wave sleep. J Clin Sleep Med. 2009; 5(6):519–524

[3] Shteamer JW, Dedhia RC. Sedative choice in drug-induced sleep endoscopy: A neuropharmacology-based review. Laryngoscope. 2017; 127(1):273–279

[4] Doherty LS, Nolan P, McNicholas WT. Effects of topical anesthesia on upper airway resistance during wake-sleep transitions. J Appl Physiol (1985). 2005; 99(2):549–555

[5] Rabelo FAW, Küpper DS, Sander HH, Fernandes RM, Valera FC. Polysomnographic evaluation of propofol-induced sleep in patients with respiratory sleep disorders and controls. Laryngoscope. 2013; 123 (9):2300–2305

[6] Gregório MG, Jacomelli M, Inoue D, Genta PR, de Figueiredo AC, Lorenzi-Filho G. Comparison of full versus short induced-sleep polysomnography for the diagnosis of sleep apnea. Laryngoscope. 2011; 121(5):1098–1103

[7] Murphy M, Bruno MA, Riedner BA, et al. Propofol anesthesia and sleep: a high-density EEG study. Sleep (Basel). 2011; 34(3):283–91A

[8] Griffin CE, III, Kaye AM, Bueno FR, Kaye AD. Benzodiazepine pharmacology and central nervous system mediated effects. Ochsner J. 2013; 13(2):214–223

[9] Forster A, Gardaz JP, Suter PM, Gemperle M. Respiratory depression by midazolam and diazepam. Anesthesiology. 1980; 53(6):494–497

[10] Genta PR, Eckert DJ, Gregório MG, et al. Critical closing pressure during midazolam-induced sleep. J Appl Physiol (1985). 2011; 111 (5):1315–1322

[11] Huupponen E, Maksimow A, Lapinlampi P, et al. Electroencephalogram spindle activity during dexmedetomidine sedation and physiological sleep. Acta Anaesthesiol Scand. 2008; 52(2):289–294

[12] De Vito A, Agnoletti V, Berrettini S, et al. Drug-induced sleep endoscopy: conventional versus target controlled infusion techniques: a randomized controlled study. Eur Arch Otorhinolaryngol. 2011; 268 (3):457–462

[13] De Vito A, Carrasco Llatas M, Ravesloot MJ, et al. European position paper on drug-induced sleep endoscopy: 2017 Update. Clin Otolaryngol. 2018; 43(6):1541–1552

10 An Anesthesiological Point of View

R.M. Corso, Massimiliano Sorbello, and Ida Di Giacinto

Abstract

Drug-induced sleep endoscopy (DISE) represents the most widespread diagnostic tool for dynamic upper airway (UA) endoscopic evaluation. The results are still debatable, and this situation calls for the need for collaboration between anesthesia, sleep medicine, and surgical providers to find safe and reliable strategies for diagnosis and treatment of airway collapse. Future research needs to look for a more thorough understanding of sedative hypnotics and their impact on airway collapsibility and sleep architecture, precise drug delivery systems, and tailored depth of sedation or anesthesia monitoring.

Keywords: obstructive sleep apnea syndrome, preoperative assessment, perioperative care, postoperative management, airway management

10.1 Introduction

Obstructive sleep apnea (OSA) is the most common form of sleep-disordered breathing (SDB). It is characterized by repetitive partial (i.e., *hypopnea*) or complete (i.e., *apnea*) collapse of the upper airway (UA) during sleep.[1] Number of these events per hour recorded during polysomnography (PSG) (apnea–hypopnea index, AHI) is commonly adopted for diagnosis and severity stratification of OSA. However, conventional measures of OSA severity do not correlate well with the severity of clinical symptoms.[2] Patients with OSA are at a higher perioperative risk due to potential difficult airway management, perioperative respiratory complications, and associated cardiovascular comorbidities.[3] Although noninvasive continuous positive airway pressure (nCPAP) is the goldstandard treatment in severe OSA, in many patients an alternative therapy, by surgery or dental appliance, is required. In these cases, the precise location of the obstruction site or sites (soft palate, lateral pharyngeal wall [LPW], tonsils, tongue base, and/or epiglottis) is critical for treatment success.[4] Drug-induced sleep endoscopy (DISE) represents the most widespread diagnostic tool for dynamic UA endoscopic evaluation, targeting possible obstruction sites.[5] The increasing evidence of the safety and utility of this technique to determine the surgical approaches has contributed to its spread, increasing the likelihood that the anesthesiologist is called to perform it.

10.2 General Anesthesia, Sedation and Sleep: Similarities and Differences

Human beings spend about one third of their lives asleep, in an active process generated by our own brain which is considered to be vital for the maintenance of health.[6] Sleep and anesthesia are two different states of consciousness, but with numerous traits in common. Similar to sleep, anesthesia represents a state of loss of consciousness, little or no recall of surrounding events, and intentional (or behavioral) immobility.[7] On the other hand, neither is anesthesia a spontaneous phenomenon, nor does it follow circadian rhythms or homeostatic processes; above all, sleep is an endogenous process, which could be easily reverted and that does not produce insensitivity to painful stimulation, differently from a (well-performed) anesthesia. Other interesting common point between anesthesia and sleep is that both are "induced": the first by a well-trained anesthesiologist, and the second by an homeostatic and circadian process actively generated in our brain, meaning that sleep is not merely not being awake, but a physiological phenomenon with biological, although not completely understood, functions such as memory retention and experience development.[8] A better understanding of sleep and anesthesia came with extensive application of electroencephalography, which allowed identification of the rapid eye movement (REM) and non-REM sleep phases with anatomical and behavioral correspondences.[9] Further biochemical findings also identified a potential role for gamma-amino-butyric acid (GABA) in receptorial modulation of REM/non-REM transitions and control of sleep/wakefulness cycle.[10] Similar electroencephalographic and biomolecular patterns have been observed during anesthesia, which has many points in common with non-REM sleep as well as some important differences. First, sleep is endogenous, hormone-regulated, and does not produce absence of response to sensory–motor or noxious stimulation; finally, the neurophysiology of general anesthesia does not show cyclic patterns of cortical deactivation/activation, but a stable plateau once anesthetic drugs reach their steadystate. GABA system has been as well called for involvement in anesthetic phenomena, whereas a growing body of literature suggests that a neuronal network with interaction among multiple neurotransmitters, rather than a single locus or molecule, should be identified as target of anesthetic action.[11] Interestingly, studies demonstrated that anesthesia is not a surrogate for sleep, whereas research on rats showed that no sleep debt had accrued during the time under anesthesia, with evidence that different anesthetics result in different sleep patterns after exposure.[12] A remarkable point is that both sleep and sensitivity to anesthesia are ubiquitous phenomena in the animal kingdom, suggesting that both of them might be someway related through mechanisms and associations which still remain largely unknown.

10.3 Anesthetics and Upper Airway

A further important common point between sleep and anesthesia is their effect on UA patency. It is a well-known phenomenon that the UA often collapses or obstructs during sedation and anesthesia. The transition to unconsciousness is typically accompanied by rapid reduction of UA muscle activity and increase in UA collapsibility.[13] Similar obstruction has been observed also during sleep: the UA is partly or completely obstructed more than 10 times per hour in about 5% of women and 15% of men in a population of individuals ranging between 30 to 60 years.[14] This event is more frequently observed during REM sleep, probably because this is phase when protective arousal responses and muscular tone and activity is on the lowest level;[15] also, nerve activity, including hypoglossal[16] and phrenic nerve,[17] sleeping position (and not merely for gravity effect on tongue),[18] and head position.[19] Notably, all of these have been supposed to be investigated as potential targets to improve treatment of OSA patients. An elegant research, despite a small patients' sample,[15] showed that the propensity for UA collapse during general anesthesia and sleep are related, especially during REM sleep, suggesting that observation of airway collapse tendency during anesthesia in a certain patient should explore and investigate presence of SDB. When focusing on airway collapse during "artificial" sleep induced by sedation or anesthesia, we should consider that a precise landmark separates a state of moderate or light sedation (*conscious sedation*) and the condition of deep sedation (and anesthesia). In the first condition, airway protecting reflexes (which we have been more focused on) are effective, and muscular tone and arousability keep a certain airway patency. In the latter case, absence of muscular tone and response produces quite often a certain degree of UA patency restriction. This dichotomy is extremely important when planning a safe sedation, with implication on importance of monitoring and assessing sedation, especially in airways with particular vulnerability to obstruction, such as those from SDB patients.[20] This is because sedation and anesthesia are a kind of "one-way" street with respect to reversibility; a fundamental difference between sleep and anesthesia is the ability of a (also)

moderate stimulation to revert to consciousness (and to airway patency and reflexes). Enhancement of tonic and phasic neuronal activation during wakefulness state provides the physiologic mechanism, granting airway tone and patency, and the loss of such an activation results in airway collapse, ending up in significant obstruction in predisposed, unprotected individuals.[21]

Degree of obstruction depends on the following factors:
- Posture: Supine position, mouth open, and neck flexed being negative factors.
- Profound muscle relaxation: sedation, anesthesia, or REM sleep.
- Airway caliber: The smaller the airway, the less the cross-section and the proportional reduction. According to Laplace's law, the smaller section results in higher transmural pressure, adding increased resistance and compliance.
- Transluminal pressure gradient: Increased with obesity, edema, and skeletal structure (micro- or retrognathia) with implications for inspiratory flow.
- Airway wall compliance: The more the compliance of an airway (meaning a soft, flaccid airway), the higher the degree of obstruction when muscular tone is lost. This also underlines role of bone and connective structures surrounding the airway in terms of maintaining a longitudinal tension.
- Muscular activation: Pharyngeal dilator muscles, the genioglossus being the most important, are controlled by hypoglossal nerve and mechanic reflex arch, whose activity is suppressed or blunt during sedation or anesthesia.

The complex architecture of UA is made out of a framework of bone and cartilage with soft tissue structures, starting from above with the nose and lips and ending at the larynx. Any "not reinforced" or particularly flaccid segment of the airway is prone to collapse once muscular tone is diminished or abolished, and typical obstruction/collapse might occur in many sites all along the UA. The velopharynx is one of the most common site of collapse during sleep and also during anesthesia, independently by depth of anesthesia but in different degrees, depending upon chosen drug and its dose. Adding of paralyzing agent might produce a further narrowing at level of hypopharynx because of a retrolingual collapse.[22] In different studies, subanesthetic doses of halothane, pentobarbital, thiopenthal, diazepam, isoflurane,[23] and propofol[24] produce different and dose-dependent degrees of airway obstruction.[13,25] Ketamine has variable effects,[26] while opioids exert a lower peripheral effect,[26] while influencing central respiratory drive.[27] If midazolam was the sedative used in the first DISE procedure carried out in 1991 by Croft and Pringle,[28] a long way has been traversed in terms of obtaining knowledge of the correlation between drugs and central nervous system and respiratory system,[29] mode of drugs administration, in association or alone, as well as the introduction, in clinical practice, of new molecules. Midazolam powerfully reduces UA muscular activity, with implications for sedation;[26] a promising drug with sedative effect and minor interference with UA muscular activity and airway collapse seems to be represented by dexmedetomidine, whereas further studies are needed to assess its safety and efficacy.[30,31] An exhaustive review of drug effects and patients' risk factors is provided by Hillman and colleagues.[13] Midazolam is usually administered as intravenous (IV) bolus, whereas propofol in continuous infusion (or, preferably, in target-controlled infusion [TCI]) represents the drug and the method of choice, as recently defined by the European Working Group.[32] Propofol bolus or ramp infusion are less performing and discouraged, nevertheless there is still heterogenicity and variability in the mode of administration and appropriate dosage of the drugs.[33] Remifentanil or ketamine are often associated with the administration of propofol and/or midazolam, taking into account the increased risks of adverse events such as desaturation. In obese patients, the administration of these drugs is even more critical because of their pharmacokinetic and pharmacodynamic properties. The growth of OSA is incremental to that of body mass index (BMI), with a higher incidence in the android distribution: dosing drugs among obese patients results in a clinical challenge, with the need for accurate and temporal monitoring in early recognition and treatment of adverse events.[34,35] TCI with propofol is unpredictable in terms of effects, and not accurate in concentration, especially in extremely high BMI. Further studies are required in the use of the ramp approach,[36] while probably remaining the best propofol administration mode among obese patients, which represent a category at relative risk during the DISE procedure.[32]

10.4 How to Monitor Sedation

Standardized protocols and safety approaches represent the gold standard in the effectiveness of DISE.[37] If the patient's essential anesthesiological monitoring is peripheral oxygen saturation (SpO$_2$), noninvasive blood pressure (NIBP) and electrocardiogram (ECG), the most critical issue when aiming for a moderate sedation is the rigorous control of dosing and an adequate feedback from monitoring depth of sedation. This assumption is of paramount importance when referring to patients with easily collapsible airways or with SDB.[38] The BIS uses electrodes placed on the forehead which monitor, through an algorithmic computation, the electroencephalographic tracing that is modified according to the administration of the drugs (this can be used with propofol and midazolam but not, for example, with ketamine). During the procedure, BIS should be between 80 and 60.[32] (▶ Fig. 10.1) SDB patients, particularly, might show unpredictability and dramatically high degrees of airway obstruction, even with moderate sedation at different levels

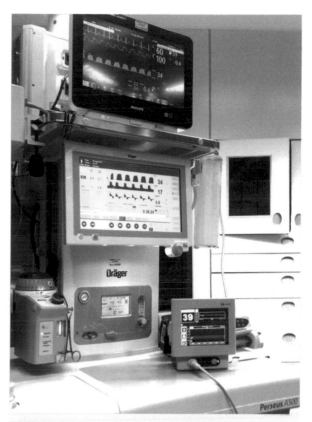

Fig. 10.1 The bispectral index brain monitoring during general anesthesia

(velopharynx, oropharynx, hypopharynx, and larynx obstructions in 77.8%, 63.3%, 30%, and 33.3% of cases respectively).[39] The same study demonstrated a linear correlation between BIS levels and grade of obstruction, offering at the same time a model of prediction and a tool to assess when level of sedation might become dangerous in terms of risk of airway collapse. Despite well-known BIS limitations,[40] it seems important to provide an objective assessment of sedation depth; entropy monitoring and/or TCI have been proposed as alternatives,[41] aiming to provide an objective method of sedation delivery. Such a result might be obtained with clinical scale or scores such as ASA continuum of sedation, modified observer's assessment of alertness/sedation scale (MOASS), and Ramsay sedation scale (RSS). Electroencephalographic processing includes BIS and entropy; alternative monitors such as the anesthesia responsiveness monitoring have been developed, which is a gold standard still missing.[42] Monitoring of capnography remains another critical point: it cannot be considered as a direct monitoring of sedation depth, but rather surrogate information. Modifications of exhaled CO_2 would provide vital information on respiratory drive and/or airway collapse, preventing adequate gas exchange. Capnography may not provide differential diagnosis for cause of hypoventilation, but it would provide fast and valuable information on patients' respiratory activity much earlier than desaturation, as detected by peripheral oxygen saturimetry, might occur.[43]

10.5 Propofol and TCI Technology

A TCI is an infusion controlled in such manner, so as to attempt to achieve a defined drug concentration in a tissue of interest. This concept was first suggested by Krüger-Thiemer in 1968.[44] This technology uses some pharmacokinetic models to predict the blood concentration of a drug after a bolus dose or after an infusion. Using this model, a computer continuously calculates the patient's expected drug concentration, adjusting pump infusion rates. Since it has been recognized that pharmacokinetics of most anesthetic agents conform best to a three-compartmental model, numerous algorithms for targeting blood and effect site concentrations have been published and several automated systems have been developed. The TCI pumps have three superimposed infusions, one infusion at a constant rate to replace drug elimination and two exponentially decreasing infusions to match drug removed from the central compartment to other peripheral compartments of distribution. The Schnider model is the most widespread pharmacokinetic model for propofol.[45] It requires age, height, and total body weight to be input for programming. The pump calculates the lean body mass for that patient and calculates doses and infusion rates accordingly. The Schnider model can only be recommended for use in effect-site targeting mode in many instances; indeed, the bolus is inappropriately small and results in an inadequate clinical effect. Older models like the Marsh model, which used the total body weight, can significantly overdose patients if actual body weights are used in obese patients. A recently described model promises improved utility in propofol administration.[46] This new model can be used in patients aged 3 months to 88 years and weighing 5 to 160 kg, solving the never ending story of weight adjustment.

10.6 Difficult Airway in OSA: Prediction and Management Strategy

Difficult airway (DA) management, combining difficult mask as well as difficult tracheal intubation, may be common in OSA patients.[47,48] Airway strategies also need to be tailored, considering morbid obesity is often associated with severe OSA. The key to safely manage the airway in the OSA patient lies in the ability to predict the difficulty and a strategy that includes multiple exit routes if needed. As a matter of fact, in case of severe predicted DA (e.g., for reduced interincisor gap precluding the insertion of a supraglottic airway device [SAD]), the indication to DISE will be revised; as in the case of complete obstruction with oxygen desaturation, the airway cannot be rescued. Recent data show that this concept is still unclear and not widespread between anesthesiologists and, even more, between the other caregivers (surgeons or nurses), who should act as a team.[49] With such premises, and due to the well-known limitations of the science in predicting a DA,[50] we strongly support a pathway strategy based on a patient-tailored approach. Such an approach should promote the idea that any airway risk should be alerted by an examination based on multiple tests,[51] any level of difficulty (difficult ventilation, laryngoscopy, SAD placement and cricothyrotomy), inclusion of nonanatomical evaluations, resources and devices availability, and team composition. This approach might probably result in overestimation of difficulties, but the filtering role of a multileveled predicting approach will dramatically reduce the incidence of unexpected critically DAs and, consequently, critical accidents. What we should aim to is not to predict only the difficult cases, but plan (every) airway crisis management, with the elaboration of a safety pathway being the main goal of any prediction strategy. Moving the target to our only objective, that is, from airway control (whichever the mean) to patients' oxygenation (▶ Fig. 10.2).

10.6.1 Face Mask Ventilation and SADs

Difficult mask ventilation is definitively difficult to predict, as recently shown in a large cohort retrospective study on a Danish database.[50] Data from literature however suggest that it occurs more often in OSA patients and that it might be associated with difficult laryngoscopy.[52] This last assumption calls for early access to SADs to rescue the airway in case of severe desaturation during DISE. SADs were introduced in clinical practice in the early 1990's with Dr. Brain's laryngeal mask airway, and since then a fast and variable evolution has been observed.[53] Data from ASA Closed Claims project[54] actually demonstrated a life-saving role of SADs during difficult/failed intubation and ventilation, acting as bridge to spontaneous ventilation or alternative techniques. NAP4[55] clearly demonstrated advantages of the so-called second generation SADs, providing gastric access and better sealing, so that nowadays no DA cart should miss a SAD, hopefully a second generation one[56] (▶ Fig. 10.3).

10.6.2 Direct Laryngoscopy versus Videolaryngoscopy

Direct laryngoscopy is used to ensure a definitive airway and can be aided by the use of a gum elastic bougie or an intubating malleable stylet, when suboptimal glottic views are obtained. Recently, videolaryngoscopy has definitely won its place in clinical practice[57,58,59] (▸ Fig. 10.4). Avoiding the need to align oral and pharyngeal axes, videolaryngoscopes (VLs) convert a difficult view through an easy procedure. It should be kept in mind that although

VLs improve glottis visualization, which is usually at the expense of prolonged tracheal intubation and does not necessarily translate into easier intubation. Today, no single VL has shown superiority with regard to its use in the OSA patient, and research to identify predictive factors of difficult videolaryngoscopy is just beginning.[60] In conclusion, patients with OSA have potentially DAs and the anesthesiologist must always be prepared for the worst-case scenario.

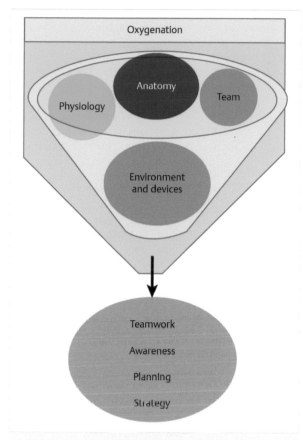

Fig. 10.2 The concept of *oxygen funnel* in predicting airway management.

10.7 Perioperative Care

Good communication between the surgeon and the anesthesia team is the key to success. It is preferable to have a dedicated anesthesiological team that understands the goal of DISE. Snoring, which leads to witnessed OSA, is the goal of DISE, and it should not be feared by the anesthesiologist. Desaturations are expected and should be tolerated. The saturation nadir or the oxygen desaturation index (ODI) recorded during sleep studies represent a useful guide to establish a reasonable threshold for desaturation. We must not forget the sleep studies are usually conducted without supplemental oxygen, sedation, or personnel skilled in airway rescue; OSA patients experience obstructive episodes and desaturations continually in their own bed. A reasonable benchmark for a safe DISE protocol would be low likelihood of severe desaturation below the sleep nadir, with rare need for airway rescue or aborted procedures.[36] In contrast to invasive procedures, DISE is a short and little invasive process, which is associated with rapid recovery profile, not necessitating inpatient admission for monitoring.[5] In our outpatient endoscopy setting, the patients undergo DISE in a series, meaning one patient comes in for DISE as the last patient goes back out to the recovery room (RR). In this area, the patients receive adequate monitoring and surveillance; the observation of recurring respiratory events in RR is an indicator to determine the need

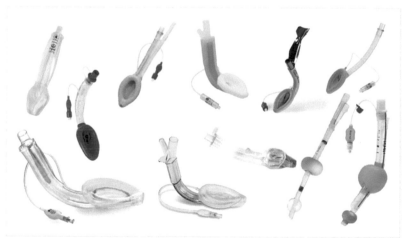

Fig. 10.3 Second generation supraglottic airway devices.

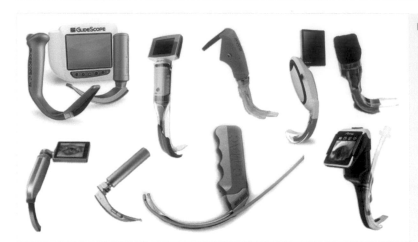

Fig. 10.4 Videolaryngoscopes.

for continuous postoperative monitoring and hospital admission.[61] The importance of the patient's position in bed must not be underestimated. A 30° position during the patient's stay in the RR and in the ward increases UA stability.[62]

10.8 Special Considerations in Pediatric Population

SDB is an epidemic in the pediatric population with a prevalence ranging from 1.2 to 5.7% but with a far greater morbidity and mortality.[63] Although adenotonsillar hypertrophy is considered as the most common cause of pediatric OSA, the obstructive mechanism is often multifactorial. In children who do not have large tonsils on initial examination, posttonsillectomy (TA) persistent OSA, or those considered to be at high risk for residual OSA after TA (patients with severe OSA, obesity, Down syndrome, craniofacial syndromes, or neuromuscular disorders), DISE can diagnose areas of obstruction in the UA other than the tonsils or adenoids guiding the treatment. DISE has no specific contraindications as long as children can undergo anesthesia;[64] however, specific competence in pediatric anesthesia is recommended.[65] In our department, patients undergo DISE in the supine position with no pillow under the head and neutral positioning. For children who require an initial mask induction for IV catheter placement, inhaled sevoflurane is used and then immediately discontinued after the catheter is placed. Propofol is then administered by TCI pump to achieve the adequate sedation level. At the end of the procedure, the child is monitored in the RR area and then admitted to pediatric surgery ward for one night. The choice of anesthetic agents for pediatric DISE is however controversial. Propofol, indeed, has been criticized for its potential to cause excessive muscle relaxation and airway collapse, which are events feared by anesthesiologists. The dose-dependent effects of propofol on the UA may manifest as

narrowing uniformly throughout the pharyngeal airway in infants and at the level of the epiglottis in older children, making the interpretation of DISE difficult.[27] A combination of dexmedetomidine and ketamine is preferred by many anesthesiologists due to the lower risk of respiratory depression and UA obstruction; however, it is characterized by a slightly longer onset of action (5–10 minutes), and patients take longer timing to recover. Regardless, further studies are needed before suggesting it as a standard sedative agent for pediatric DISE.[66] In addition to these agents, most children require inhalational anesthetic in order to insert an IV line. Because inhalational anesthetics have been shown to decrease UA muscle activity and confound findings during DISE,[67] it is recommended that inhalational agents be discontinued as soon as IV access is obtained and DISE delayed until the agent is out.[68]

10.9 Conclusion

A patient affected by obstructive sleep apnea syndrome (OSAS) undergoing DISE is a patient at high risk from adverse events in the perioperative phase which can be avoided only by the implementation of a well-defined clinical pathway. Good communication between anesthesia providers and surgeons is also particularly important, as patients with OSA are at greater risk of airway obstruction and oxygen desaturation when sedated, and oversedation can result in airway compromise and/or central apnea.

Note: The authors declare that there are no conflicts of interest.

References

[1] Jordan AS, McSharry DG, Malhotra A. Adult obstructive sleep apnoea. Lancet. 2014; 383(9918):736–747
[2] Randerath W, Bassetti CL, Bonsignore MR, et al. Challenges and perspectives in obstructive sleep apnoea: report by an ad hoc working

group of the Sleep Disordered Breathing Group of the European Respiratory Society and the European Sleep Research Society. Eur Respir J. 2018; 52(3):1702616

[3] Corso R, Russotto V, Gregoretti C, Cattano D. Perioperative management of obstructive sleep apnea: a systematic review. Minerva Anestesiol. 2018; 84(1):81–93

[4] MacKay SG, Chan L. Surgical approaches to obstructive sleep apnea. Sleep Med Clin. 2016, 11(3):331–341

[5] De Vito A, Carrasco Llatas M, Vanni A, et al. European position paper on drug-induced sedation endoscopy (DISE). Sleep Breath. 2014; 18 (3):453–465

[6] Brown EN, Lydic R, Schiff ND. General anesthesia, sleep, and coma. N Engl J Med. 2010; 363(27):2638–2650

[7] Sejnowski TJ, Destexhe A. Why do we sleep? Brain Res. 2000; 886 (1–2):208–223

[8] Oishi Y, Lazarus M. The control of sleep and wakefulness by mesolimbic dopamine systems. Neurosci Res. 2017; 118:66–73

[9] Aserinsky E, Kleitman N. Regularly occurring periods of eye motility, and concomitant phenomena, during sleep. Science. 1953; 118 (3062):273–274

[10] Hassani OK, Henny P, Lee MG, Jones BE. GABAergic neurons intermingled with orexin and MCH neurons in the lateral hypothalamus discharge maximally during sleep. Eur J Neurosci. 2010; 32(3): 448–457

[11] Vanini G, Watson CJ, Lydic R, Baghdoyan HA. Gamma-aminobutyric acid-mediated neurotransmission in the pontine reticular formation modulates hypnosis, immobility, and breathing during isoflurane anesthesia. Anesthesiology. 2008; 109(6):978–988

[12] Tung A, Lynch JP, Mendelson WB. Prolonged sedation with propofol in the rat does not result in sleep deprivation. Anesth Analg. 2001; 92 (5):1232–1236

[13] Hillman DR, Platt PR, Eastwood PR. The upper airway during anaesthesia. Br J Anaesth. 2003; 91(1):31–39

[14] Young T, Palta M, Dempsey J, Skatrud J, Weber S, Badr S. The occurrence of sleep-disordered breathing among middle-aged adults. N Engl J Med. 1993; 328(17):1230–1235

[15] Eastwood PR, Szollosi I, Platt PR, Hillman DR. Comparison of upper airway collapse during general anaesthesia and sleep. Lancet. 2002; 359(9313):1207–1209

[16] Heiser C, Hofauer B. [Stimulation for sleep apnea. targeting the hypoglossal nerve in the treatment of patients with OSA]. HNO. 2018; 66 (9):705–716

[17] Hillman DR, Walsh JH, Maddison KJ, Platt PR, Schwartz AR, Eastwood PR. The effect of diaphragm contraction on upper airway collapsibility. J Appl Physiol (1985). 2013; 115(3):337–345

[18] Marques M, Genta PR, Sands SA, et al. Effect of sleeping position on upper airway patency in obstructive sleep apnea is determined by the pharyngeal structure causing collapse. Sleep (Basel). 2017; 40(3)

[19] Walsh JH, Maddison KJ, Platt PR, Hillman DR, Eastwood PR. Influence of head extension, flexion, and rotation on collapsibility of the passive upper airway. Sleep. 2008; 31(10):1440–1447

[20] Hillman DR, Platt PR, Eastwood PR. Anesthesia, sleep, and upper airway collapsibility. Anesthesiol Clin. 2010; 28(3):443–455

[21] Hillman DR, Loadsman JA, Platt PR, Eastwood PR. Obstructive sleep apnoea and anaesthesia. Sleep Med Rev. 2004; 8(6):459–471

[22] Mathru M, Esch O, Lang J, et al. Magnetic resonance imaging of the upper airway. Effects of propofol anesthesia and nasal continuous positive airway pressure in humans. Anesthesiology. 1996; 84(2):273–279

[23] Eastwood PR, Szollosi I, Platt PR, Hillman DR. Collapsibility of the upper airway during anesthesia with isoflurane. Anesthesiology. 2002; 97(4):786–793

[24] Eastwood PR, Platt PR, Shepherd K, Maddison K, Hillman DR. Collapsibility of the upper airway at different concentrations of propofol anesthesia. Anesthesiology. 2005; 103(3):470–477

[25] Hillman DR, Walsh JH, Maddison KJ, et al. Evolution of changes in upper airway collapsibility during slow induction of anesthesia with propofol. Anesthesiology. 2009; 111(1):63–71

[26] Drummond GB. Comparison of sedation with midazolam and ketamine: effects on airway muscle activity. Br J Anaesth. 1996; 76 (5):663–667

[27] Ehsan Z, Mahmoud M, Shott SR, Amin RS, Ishman SL. The effects of anesthesia and opioids on the upper airway: a systematic review. Laryngoscope. 2016; 126(1):270–284

[28] Croft CB, Pringle M. Sleep nasendoscopy: a technique of assessment in snoring and obstructive sleep apnoea. Clin Otolaryngol Allied Sci. 1991; 16(5):504–509

[29] Blumen M, Bequignon E, Chabolle F. Drug-induced sleep endoscopy: a new gold standard for evaluating OSAS? Part I: Technique. Eur Ann Otorhinolaryngol Head Neck Dis. 2017; 134(2):101–107

[30] Shteamer JW, Dedhia RC. Sedative choice in drug-induced sleep endoscopy: A neuropharmacology-based review. Laryngoscope. 2017; 127(1):273–279

[31] Chang ET, Certal V, Song SA, et al. Dexmedetomidine versus propofol during drug-induced sleep endoscopy and sedation: a systematic review. Sleep Breath. 2017; 21(3):727–735

[32] De Vito A, Carrasco Llatas M, Ravesloot MJ, et al. European position paper on drug-induced sleep endoscopy: 2017 Update. Clin Otolaryngol. 2018; 43(6):1541–1552

[33] Atkins JH, Mandel JE. Drug-induced sleep endoscopy: from obscure technique to diagnostic tool for assessment of obstructive sleep apnea for surgical interventions. Curr Opin Anaesthesiol. 2018; 31 (1):120–126

[34] Lechner M, Wilkins D, Kotecha B. A review on drug-induced sedation endoscopy: technique, grading systems and controversies. Sleep Med Rev. 2018; 41:141–148

[35] Petrini F, Di Giacinto I, Cataldo R, et al. Obesity Task Force for the SIAARTI Airway Management Study Group. Perioperative and periprocedural airway management and respiratory safety for the obese patient: 2016 SIAARTI Consensus. Minerva Anestesiol. 2016; 82(12): 1314–1335

[36] Atkins JH, Mandel JE, Rosanova G. Safety and efficacy of drug-induced sleep endoscopy using a probability ramp propofol infusion system in patients with severe obstructive sleep apnea. Anesth Analg. 2014; 119(4):805–810

[37] Dijemeni E, D'Amone G. Is sedation administration strategy and analysis during drug induced sedation endoscopy objective and systematic? Sleep Breath. 2018; 22(1):181–182

[38] Memtsoudis SG, Cozowicz C, Nagappa M, et al. Society of Anesthesia and Sleep Medicine guideline on intraoperative management of adult patients with obstructive sleep apnea. Anesth Analg. 2018; 127(4): 967–987

[39] Lo YL, Ni YL, Wang TY, et al. Bispectral index in evaluating effects of sedation depth on drug-induced sleep endoscopy. J Clin Sleep Med. 2015; 11(9):1011–1020

[40] Stierer TL, Ishman SL. Bispectral index in evaluating effects of sedation depth on drug-induced sleep endoscopy: DISE or no dice. J Clin Sleep Med. 2015; 11(9):965–966

[41] Heiser C, Fthenakis P, Hapfelmeier A, et al. Drug-induced sleep endoscopy with target-controlled infusion using propofol and monitored depth of sedation to determine treatment strategies in obstructive sleep apnea. Sleep Breath. 2017; 21(3):737–744

[42] Sheahan CG, Mathews DM. Monitoring and delivery of sedation. Br J Anaesth. 2014; 113 Suppl 2:ii37–ii47

[43] Conway A, Douglas C, Sutherland J. Capnography monitoring during procedural sedation and analgesia: a systematic review protocol. Syst Rev. 2015; 4:92

[44] Krüger-Thiemer E. Continuous intravenous infusion and multicompartment accumulation. Eur J Pharmacol. 1968; 4(3):317–324

[45] Sahinovic MM, Struys MMRF, Absalom AR. Clinical pharmacokinetics and pharmacodynamics of propofol. Clin Pharmacokinet. 2018; 57 (12):1539–1558

[46] Eleveld DJ, Proost JH, Cortínez LI, Absalom AR, Struys MM. A general purpose pharmacokinetic model for propofol. Anesth Analg. 2014; 118(6):1221–1237

[47] Corso RM, Petrini F, Buccioli M, et al. Clinical utility of preoperative screening with STOP-Bang questionnaire in elective surgery. Minerva Anestesiol. 2014; 80(8):877–884

[48] Cattano D, Killoran PV, Cai C, Katsiampoura AD, Corso RM, Hagberg CA. Difficult mask ventilation in general surgical population: observation of risk factors and predictors. F1000 Res. 2014; 3:204

[49] Corso RM, Sorbello M, Buccioli M, et al. Survey of knowledge and attitudes about obstructive sleep apnoea among Italian anaesthetists. Turk J Anaesthesiol Reanim. 2017; 45(3):146–152

[50] Nørskov AK, Rosenstock CV, Wetterslev J, Astrup G, Afshari A, Lundstrøm LH. Diagnostic accuracy of anaesthesiologists' prediction of difficult airway management in daily clinical practice: a cohort study of 188 064 patients registered in the Danish Anaesthesia Database. Anaesthesia. 2015; 70(3):272–281

[51] Corso RM, Cattano D, Buccioli M, Carretta E, Maitan S. [Post analysis simulated correlation of the El-Ganzouri airway difficulty score with difficult airway]. Rev Bras Anestesiol. 2016; 66(3):298–303

[52] Leong SM, Tiwari A, Chung F, Wong DT. Obstructive sleep apnea as a risk factor associated with difficult airway management: a narrative review. J Clin Anesth. 2018; 45:63–68

[53] Sorbello M. Evolution of supraglottic airway devices: the Darwinian perspective. Minerva Anestesiol. 2018; 84(3):297–300

[54] Metzner J, Posner KL, Lam MS, Domino KB. Closed claims' analysis. Best Pract Res Clin Anaesthesiol. 2011; 25(2):263–276

[55] Cook TM, Woodall N, Frerk C, Fourth National Audit Project. Major complications of airway management in the UK: results of the Fourth National Audit Project of the Royal College of Anaesthetists and the Difficult Airway Society. Part 1: anaesthesia. Br J Anaesth. 2011; 106 (5):617–631

[56] Cook TM, Kelly FE. Time to abandon the 'vintage' laryngeal mask airway and adopt second-generation supraglottic airway devices as first choice. Br J Anaesth. 2015; 115(4):497–499

[57] Wilson WM, Smith AF. The emerging role of awake videolaryngoscopy in airway management. Anaesthesia. 2018; 73(9):1058–1061

[58] Alhomary M, Ramadan E, Curran E, Walsh SR. Videolaryngoscopy vs. fibreoptic bronchoscopy for awake tracheal intubation: a systematic review and meta-analysis. Anaesthesia. 2018; 73(9): 1151–1161

[59] Cook TM, Boniface NJ, Seller C, et al. Universal videolaryngoscopy: a structured approach to conversion to videolaryngoscopy for all intubations in an anaesthetic and intensive care department. Br J Anaesth. 2018; 120(1):173–180

[60] Hoshijima H, Denawa Y, Tominaga A, Nakamura C, Shiga T, Nagasaka H. Videolaryngoscope versus Macintosh laryngoscope for tracheal intubation in adults with obesity: A systematic review and meta-analysis. J Clin Anesth. 2018; 44:69–75

[61] Gali B, Whalen FX, Schroeder DR, Gay PC, Plevak DJ. Identification of patients at risk for postoperative respiratory complications using a preoperative obstructive sleep apnea screening tool and postanesthesia care assessment. Anesthesiology. 2009; 110(4): 869–877

[62] Neill AM, Angus SM, Sajkov D, McEvoy RD. Effects of sleep posture on upper airway stability in patients with obstructive sleep apnea. Am J Respir Crit Care Med. 1997; 155(1):199–204

[63] Marcus CL, Brooks LJ, Draper KA, et al. American Academy of Pediatrics. Diagnosis and management of childhood obstructive sleep apnea syndrome. Pediatrics. 2012; 130(3):e714–e755

[64] Charakorn N, Kezirian EJ. Drug-induced sleep endoscopy. Otolaryngol Clin North Am. 2016; 49(6):1359–1372

[65] Disma N, Calderini E, SIAARTI-SARNePI Committee on Paediatric Anaesthesia. SIAARTI-SARNePI clinical-organizational standards for pediatric anesthesia. Minerva Anestesiol. 2018; 84(2):143–146

[66] Kandil A, Subramanyam R, Hossain MM, et al. Comparison of the combination of dexmedetomidine and ketamine to propofol or propofol/sevoflurane for drug-induced sleep endoscopy in children. Paediatr Anaesth. 2016; 26(7):742–751

[67] Friedman NR, Parikh SR, Ishman SL, et al. The current state of pediatric drug-induced sleep endoscopy. Laryngoscope. 2017; 127 (1):266–272

[68] Galluzzi F, Pignataro L, Gaini RM, Garavello W. Drug induced sleep endoscopy in the decision-making process of children with obstructive sleep apnea. Sleep Med. 2015; 16(3):331–335

11 Work in Progress: A Prediction Model for DISE as Selection Tool for MAD and Positional Therapy

Patty E. Vonk, Annemieke M.E.H. Beelen, and Nico de Vries

Abstract

To evaluate the effect of different passive maneuvers during drug-induced sleep endoscopy (DISE), a retrospective, single-center cohort study of 200 obstructive sleep apnea (OSA) patients was performed. All patients underwent DISE with and without manually performed jaw thrust and lateral head rotation by using the velum, oropharynx, tongue base and epiglottis (VOTE) classification. The model leaves room for improvement. The effect of manually performed jaw thrust is greater and the effect of lateral head rotation alone is less than what was expected compared to recent literature on treatment outcome of oral appliance theory (OAT), positional therapy (PT) and combined treatment.

Keywords: obstructive sleep apnea, drug-induced sleep endoscopy, oral device, positional therapy

11.1 Introduction

Drug-induced sleep endoscopy (DISE) is, as stated in earlier chapters, a controversial diagnostic tool. It is mostly performed by ENTs, in particular sleep surgeons. Not all sleep surgeons would agree that DISE is always mandatory in case sleep surgery is considered. Notably, ENT obstructive sleep apnea (OSA) caregivers such as pulmonologists, neurologists and maxillofacial surgeons often question the usefulness of DISE further. Even more controversial is the role of DISE in case other nonsurgical treatments and combination therapies are considered.

DISE provides information regarding the degree, level(s), and configuration of obstruction of the collapsible segment of the upper airway (UA) in case UA surgery is considered. The role of DISE is less well-explored in patients in whom other OSA treatment modalities, such as oral appliance therapy (OAT), positional therapy (PT) with new generation positional devices, combined treatment (e.g., OAT and PT), and PT after UA surgery, are considered.

Presently, in case OAT is considered, patients in most institutes are simply prescribed such a device without additional evaluation of the UA through DISE. Using this pragmatic approach, OAT is effective in 30 to 81%.[1] This implies that a considerable number of patients after a lengthy process of mandibular advancement device (MAD) production, fitting and titration will get an expensive MAD that later, subjectively and objectively, appears to be not sufficiently effective in repeat sleep study. An alternative approach would involve performing a DISE

first and mimic the effect of OAT (e.g., by performing a jaw thrust), and only embark on OAT in case the airway opens with jaw thrust. The assumption is that this would lead to a higher percentage of successful OAT. As discussed earlier, the risk of a *lege artis* performed DISE in well-selected patients is negligible, but the flip side of this approach is that DISE is time consuming and costs money. Furthermore, the positive predictive value of the performance of jaw thrust during DISE is questioned by many. Antagonists are of the opinion that by bringing the lower jaw forward most airways will indeed open, but point to the fact that jaw thrust is a very unprecise maneuver and in no way a reliable reflection of the 60 to 75% of maximum forward movement that is intended with OAT. Intuitively, the negative predictive value of jaw thrust has more meaning. Why should one even try a MAD in case obstruction, be it at the level of palate, oropharynx, base of tongue, epiglottis or more than one level, persists during DISE with maximum protrusion of the mandible?

However, even with regard to the negative predictive value of jaw thrust, little evidence is available.[2,3,4]

The research group of Antwerp, Belgium, has taken the matter to another level and studied the usefulness of simulation bites during DISE. Vroegop et al investigated the use of simulation bites and found a significant association between positive effect of the simulation bite and treatment response to OAT. Unfortunately, at this point, the use of simulation bites is even more time consuming than jaw thrust, more costly, and therefore not routinely feasible or common practice and still only used for research purposes.[5]

Similarly, in case PT is considered, it might be useful to compare DISE findings in lateral and supine position. Recent research from the groups from Antwerp and Amsterdam has shown that in mild to moderate positional OSA (POSA), the effects of OAT and PT are comparable, with roughly 50% statistically significant reduction in apnea–hypopnea index (AHI). Combined OAT and PT leads to a further 50% statistically significant reduction in AHI.[6,7,8]

Regarding the correlation between AHI and observations made during DISE, several studies point in the same direction. Vroegop et al concluded that higher AHI values are associated with a complete collapse observed during DISE, particularly a complete concentric collapse (CCC) at palatal level and a complete lateral hypopharyngeal collapse. Lower AHI was associated with a higher probability of a partial concentric collapse.[9]

Ravesloot et al found similar results and suggested that a multilevel collapse, complete collapse, and tongue base collapse are associated with a higher AHI.[10]

The department of ENT at OLVG West Hospital in Amsterdam, The Netherlands, serves as a referral center for patients who seek alternatives to continuous positive airway pressure (CPAP) treatment. Some 800 DISEs are performed annually. Since 2017, PT with new generation positional devices in mild to moderate POSA is reimbursed in The Netherlands. However, so far, combined treatment (PT and MAD), or PT in severe POSA, is not reimbursed. As a rule, in these second opinion and referral patients, we want to keep all treatment options open, and in such patients at the time of the present study: we performed DISE in four positions supine, supine with jaw thrust (to mimic the effect of OAT), lateral head rotation (to mimic the effect of PT), and jaw thrust with head rotation (to mimic combined treatment with OAT and PT).

For the study presented in this chapter,[11] we composed a 3 points model, based on the velum, oropharynx, tongue base and epiglottis (VOTE) classification system, in which the effects of these maneuvers were retrospectively analyzed. In case of a perfect fit of the model, the effect of jaw thrust and head rotation would be equal (50% reduction in points), with another 50% reduction in case of combined maneuvers.

We hypothesized that the effect of these maneuvers would correspond with recent literature on treatment outcomes of PT, OAT and combined treatment and could therefore serve as a tool in patient-specific treatment planning.[6,7,8] When our hypothesis would be correct, DISE with these maneuvers could prove to be of additional value in predicting positive or negative treatment outcome of OAT, PT or combined treatment.

11.2 Methods

11.2.1 Patients

We performed a retrospective, single-center cohort study including a consecutive series of 200 OSA patients, confirmed by polysomnography (PSG), who underwent DISE between August 2016 and February 2017. Patients were excluded from analysis when <18 years, medical history of congenital abnormalities of the UA, DISE performed with CPAP or OAT, and when DISE results were inconclusive due to mucus hypersecretion. Patients were classified as being nonpositional (NPP) or positional (PP) using a modified version of Cartwright's criteria,[12] namely, a difference of 50% or more in AHI between supine and nonsupine positions and a total sleeping time in worse sleeping position of >10% and <90%. In PP, a further distinction was made between supine isolated (nonsupine AHI < 5 event/h) and supine predominant (nonsupine AHI ≥ 5 events/h).[13] In accordance with the Declaration of Helsinki, the study protocol was approved by the Medical

Ethical Committee. Data on study subjects was collected and stored anonymously to protect personal information.

11.2.2 DISE Procedure

DISE was performed in patients in whom alternatives to CPAP were considered. We not only looked at eligibility for UA surgery, but also evaluated the possible effect of other conservative treatments such as OAT, PT or combination of both. In some patients, DISE was performed to identify reasons for previous treatment failure (e.g., OAT or CPAP).

DISE was performed in a quiet outpatient endoscopy room with dimmed lights and standard anesthetic equipment. The procedure was executed by two trained ENT residents (PV and AB), with a nurse anesthetist managing sedation. The desired level of propofol concentration was controlled by the nurse anesthetist by using a target-controlled infusion (TCI) pump. Prior to the propofol, 2 mL lidocaine was given intravenously to prevent pain caused by the infusion of propofol. On indication, glycopyrrolate was administered before the procedure to avoid excessive secretions, which may interfere with the quality of the DISE video. Propofol concentration was gradually increased until proper sedation was achieved. Proper sedation was reached when the patient began to snore or showed hyporesponsiveness to verbal and tactile stimuli. The UA was observed by using a flexible laryngoscopy, starting in supine position with and without jaw thrust. Subsequently, lateral head rotation to the right was performed again with and without jaw thrust.

11.2.3 Classification System

The VOTE system was used to evaluate four different levels and structures that can contribute to UA obstruction, namely, velum (V), oropharynx (O), tongue base (T), and epiglottis (E). The degree of obstruction was defined by the following categories: no obstruction (collapse less than 50%), partial (collapse between 50–75%, typically with vibration) or complete collapse (> 75%), and X if no observation could be made. The configuration of the obstruction may be anterior–posterior, lateral or concentric.[14] ▶ Table 11.1 shows an overview of the different levels, degree of obstruction, and possible configurations at each level.

In the present model, we regarded obstruction at the four levels equally important, but concentric collapse at velum level as more severe than lateral or anteroposterior (AP) collapse, because literature has shown that a CCC of the palate correspond with a less successful treatment outcome when applying OAT or UA surgery.[15,16] Therefore, we introduced a 3 point scale: no obstruction = 0 points; partial lateral or AP obstruction = 1 point; partial concentric obstruction at velum level = 2 points; complete

Table 11.1 The VOTE classification[14]

Structure	Degree of obstruction[a]	Configuration[c]		
		Anteroposterior	Lateral	Concentric
Velum				
Oropharynx[b]		▨		▨
Tongue base			▨	▨
Epiglottis				▨

Abbreviation: VOTE: velum, oropharynx, tongue base, and epiglottis.
[a] Degree of obstruction: 0 no obstruction; 1 partial obstruction; 2 complete obstruction.
[b] Oropharynx obstruction can be distinguished as related solely to the tonsils or including the lateral walls.
[c] Configuration noted for structures with degree of obstruction >0.

lateral or AP obstruction = 2 points; complete concentric obstruction at velum level = 4 points.

11.2.4 Statistical Analysis

Statistical analysis was performed using SPSS (version 21), SPSS Inc., Chicago, IL). Quantitative data are reported as mean ± SD or as median (Q1, Q3) when not normally distributed.

To analyze the effect of different passive maneuvers on UA caliber, the score that describes the degree of obstruction (0, 1 and 2) at the four separate structures (V, O, T and E) was used. For the comparison of overall effect of these maneuvers, the total sum VOTE score was calculated by summing the different scores for degree of obstruction at each site. The total sum VOTE score is reported as median (Q1, Q3), since it is a sum of categorical data and therefore must be analyzed as ordinal data.

Comparison of data on total sum VOTE scores in different positions, with and without maneuvers, between the different subgroups was carried out by using the Wilcoxon signed rank test in case of paired data and a chi-squared test in case of unpaired data. A p value of < 0.05 was considered to indicate statistical significance.

11.3 Results

In total, 200 patients were included in this study, of which 80.5% was male. The mean age was 50.1 ± 11.7 years, with a body mass index (BMI) of 27.0 ± 3.1 kg/m^2 and a median AHI of 19.2 events per hour. Forty-four per cent of the patients were NPP; of the remaining 56%, 34% was diagnosed with supine isolated and 66% with supine predominant POSA. As expected, PP had a significant lower AHI in nonsupine position and spent more time in supine position. Patients with supine isolated POSA showed a significantly lower total AHI, a lower AHI in supine and nonsupine position, and spent more time in

supine position compared to supine predominant PP. Baseline characteristics are given in ▶ Table 11.2 and ▶ Table 11.3.

In all subgroups, the median total sum VOTE score in supine position was 6.0 and 2.0, respectively when jaw thrust was added, which is a significant reduction of 66.7% ($p = 0.00$). In NPP and supine-predominant PP, the median total sum VOTE score of 6.0 in supine position showed a significant reduction of 2 points (33.3%) when lateral head rotation was performed ($p = 0.00$). This is in contrast to patients with supine-isolated POSA, where a significant reduction of 50% (6.0 versus 3.0) was found ($p = 0.00$). When comparing the effect of lateral head rotation in supine-isolated and supine-predominant PP, a significant difference was found in favor of the supine isolated group ($p = 0.03$). When both maneuvers were combined (lateral head rotation and jaw thrust), the median total sum VOTE score in all subgroups changed from 6.0 in supine position to 1.0 ($p = 0.00$), except for the supine isolated PP group, which showed a significant reduction to 0.5 ($p = 0.00$), but this difference was not significant when supine-isolated and supine-predominant PP were compared ($p = 0.682$).

An overview of the different total sum VOTE scores in different positions with and without maneuvers is presented in ▶ Table 11.4.

11.4 Discussion

DISE is a diagnostic tool for UA evaluation in patients diagnosed with OSA. In many cases DISE findings change patient management, and evidence is accumulating that DISE provides valuable information to predict treatment response and surgical success.[17,18] Different passive maneuvers can be performed during DISE with the intent to predict treatment response of current available treatment modalities. In the present study, we evaluated the additional value of DISE, including maneuvers for PT, OAT or a combination of both.

Table 11.2 Baseline characteristics total population and NPP versus PP

	Total	NPP	PP	NPP vs. PP p value
Number (%)	200	88 (44)	112 (56)	88 vs 112
Age (years)	50.1 ± 11.7	52.4 ± 10.8	48.2 ± 12.1	0.010[b]
Male/Female	161/39	68/20	93/19	0.307
BMI (kg/m²)	27.0 ± 3.1	27.0 ± 3.1	27.1 ± 3.2	0.832
Total AHI	19.2 (11.7, 31.0)[a]	21.0 (14.0, 38.4)[a]	18.3 (10.7, 27.3)[a]	0.073
Supine AHI	34.5 (18.4, 59.0)[a]	25.7 (15.9, 61.4)[a]	37.8 (22.6, 57.9)[a]	0.095
Nonsupine AHI	10.8 (5.4, 22.8)[a]	19.4 (9.9, 34.8)[a]	7.3 (3.4, 14.7)[a]	0.00[b]
Supine sleeping time (%)	31.5 (16.6, 50.2)[a]	21.4 (3.7, 44.4)[a]	35.4 (22.0, 50.5)[a]	0.001[b]

Abbreviations: NPP, nonpositional obstructive sleep apnea patients; PP, positional-dependent obstructive sleep apnea patients; BMI, body mass index; AHI, apnea–hypopnea index.
[a] Median (Q1, Q3); [b] p value <0.05.

Table 11.3 Baseline characteristics PP supine isolated versus PP supine predominant

N = 112	Supine isolated	Supine predominant	Supine isolated versus supine predominant p value
Number (%)	38 (34)	74 (66)	38 vs. 74
Age (years)	46.1 ± 11.0	49.2 ± 12.5	0.196
Male/Female	29/9	64/10	0.175
BMI (kg/m²)	26.3 ± 3.2	27.4 ± 3.2	0.087
Total AHI	8.8 (6.2, 16.3)[a]	23.0 (15.9, 33.3)[a]	0.00[b]
Supine AHI	19.1 (11.4, 34.0)[a]	47.7 (33.6, 63.8)[a]	0.00[b]
Non supine AHI	2.5 (1.6, 3.5)[a]	10.8 (7.4, 19.4)[a]	0.00[b]
Supine sleeping time (%)	45.0 (33.6, 64.9)[a]	30.0 (21.0, 45.5)[a]	0.002[b]

Abbreviations: PP, positional-dependent obstructive sleep apnea patients; BMI, body mass index; AHI, apnea–hypopnea index.
[a] Median (Q1, Q3); [b] p value < 0.05.

A meta-analysis performed by Ravesloot et al evaluated the effectiveness of PT in improving sleep study variables in positional OSA. The results of six studies were used for analysis and showed that total AHI was significantly reduced when PT was applied from a mean of 21.8 ± 7.2 to 9.9 ± 10.6, a difference of 53.6%.[19]

Several studies have showed that OAT is effective in both reducing AHI and decreasing OSA symptoms.[1,20] A study by Dieltjens et al prospectively evaluated the treatment response of a titratable OA. They found a success rate of 55.7%, a decrease of total AHI of more than 50% and a total AHI of less than 10. The effectiveness of

Table 11.4 Total sum VOTE score in different positions with and without maneuvers

	Total	NPP	PP	PP supine isolated	PP supine predominant
Supine	6.0 (4.0, 6.0)	6.0 (4.0, 6.0)	6.0 (4.0, 6.0)	6.0 (4.0, 6.0)	6.0 (5.0, 7.0)
Supine + jaw thrust	2.0 (1.0, 3.0)	2.0 (0.0, 2.0)	2.0 (1.0, 3.0)	2.0 (1.0, 2.0)	2.0 (1.0, 3.0)
Lateral head rotation	4.0 (3.0, 6.0)	4.0 (3.0, 6.0)	4.0 (3.0, 6.0)	3.0 (2.0, 5.5)	4.0 (3.0, 6.0)
Lateral head rotation + jaw thrust	1.0 (0.0, 2.0)	1.0 (0.0, 3.0)	1.0 (0.0, 2.0)	0.5 (0.0, 2.0)	1.0 (0.0, 2.0)

Abbreviations: NPP, nonpositional obstructive sleep apnea patients; PP, positional-dependent obstructive sleep apnea patients.
Note: Values described as median (Q1, Q3).

combined treatment with OAT + PT (with the Sleep Position Trainer of Night Balance) has also prospectively been investigated. Both OAT and PT were individually effective in reducing AHI with approximately 50%, while the combination of PT + OAT further reduced total AHI, with another 50% compared to SPT or OAT alone, leading to in total approximately 75% reduction.[8]

In the model we tested in the present study, we regarded obstruction at the four levels (velum, oropharynx, tongue base and epiglottis) as equally important, but a concentric collapse as more severe than lateral or AP collapse, since it has been shown that a CCC at palatal level corresponds to a worse treatment outcome than AP or lateral collapse. This holds true for OAT, UA surgery and upper airway stimulation (UAS). Vanderveken et al found that the overall treatment success with hypoglossal nerve stimulation in patients without a CCC at palatal level was 81%, while treatment success could not be achieved in the presence of a CCC of the palate.[16] In a study by Koutsourelakis et al for UAS surgery, similar results were found. They concluded that nonresponders to UA surgery had a higher occurrence of a CCC at palatal level compared to responders.[15]

When interpreting our results, it must be taken into account that the reduction in total sum VOTE score is calculated by summing the median score of the presence of obstruction at the four levels. Therefore, "reduction" actually must be interpreted as a left shift of the median and distribution of the data.

If our model would have been a perfect fit, the reduction by either performing the jaw thrust or head rotation would both give a 50% reduction in points. Jaw thrust, however, gave a more than 50% reduction. As expected, a 50% reduction was seen in supine-isolated PP when lateral head rotation was performed, but in contrast to what was hypothesized, a reduction of less than 50% was seen in supine-predominant PP. The difference in results between supine-isolated and supine-predominant might

be explained by the greater difference between the supine and nonsupine AHI in supine-isolated PP. Previous studies also demonstrate an important influence of head position on the AHI, independently of trunk position and sleep stage, but at this point, the effect of having supine-isolated or supine-predominant POSA needs to be further unravelled.[21,22]

The estimated 75% reduction of the combination of those two maneuvers was almost as predicted, but higher than expected by jaw thrust, probably based on the erroneously product of the overestimation of the maneuver, while the effect of head rotation was less than expected.

We performed a manual jaw thrust and tried to protrude the mandible less than 100%, aiming at roughly 50 to 75% protrusion. We are aware that this is a very unprecise maneuver. The predictive value of manually performed jaw thrust on treatment response to OAT varies between different studies. Johal et al found a good correlation between the maneuver and treatment success rate.[2,3] Eichler et al also concluded that the effect of mandibular advancement can be shown during DISE.[23] In contrast, Vanderveken et al and Vroegop et al have been questioning the correlation between the effect of the chin lift maneuver during DISE and treatment success of OAT, and suggested the use of a simulation bite during DISE, which tends to better predict response to OAT.[4,5]

The present study indeed confirms the suspicion that manual jaw thrust leads to an overestimation of an OAT effect, because in this study, we found a reduction of 66.7% when jaw thrust was added instead of the expected effect of 50%.

We previously reported two DISE studies on the effect of lateral rotation of the head alone and of both head and trunk.[24,25] These studies suggested that the effect of head rotation alone, and of head and trunk rotation combined were almost comparable in terms of level(s) and direction of obstruction. We were less convinced that the quantitative effect was equal, but for practical reasons—head rotation is much easier to carry out than head and trunk rotation combined—lateral head rotation was subsequently adopted in clinical practice. Still, we remained critical since we are aware that not all patients are capable of a full 90% head rotation.

In this study, the range of individual head rotation was not routinely tested before performing DISE. When the maximum of lateral head rotation was limited, an annotation was made, but patients were not excluded in this study. This physical limitation might lead to an underestimation of the effect of lateral head rotation. The present study confirms the suspicion that head rotation alone might provide less improvement than expected. Rotation of both head and trunk was not tested in the present study.

Overall, NPP tend to have more severe OSA compared to PP and the incidence of POSA increases when the OSA severity decreases.[26,27,28] A previous study also showed that a multilevel collapse is associated with higher AHI, and a tongue base collapse or epiglottal collapse is associated with POSA.[10] Based on these findings, one would expect a higher sum VOTE score in NPP compared to PP.

In contrast to what was expected, similar results were found in NPP and PP when comparing the sum VOTE score in different positions. We believe that this could be explained by several reasons.

First, patients undergoing DISE are usually diagnosed with mild to moderate OSA, since CPAP is still the gold-standard therapy in case of severe OSA. Therefore, DISE usually is not performed in severe OSA patients, unless they experience CPAP failure/intolerance or when UA surgery is considered. This selection in patients could influence our results, because as mentioned, the prevalence of POSA decreases as the severity of OSA increases.

Second, in our study population, no significant difference was found in total and supine AHI. Although a significant difference was found between nonsupine AHI in NPP and PP, NPP did show a lower AHI in nonsupine position. A previous study showed that head rotation only can influence UA collapsibility and improve AHI compared to supine position, whether patients are diagnosed with POSA or not.[21,22] On the other hand, it could also be possible that the effect of lateral head rotation only is too minimal to differentiate the effectiveness between NPP and PP.

11.5 Conclusion and Future Perspectives

We conclude that the present model leaves room for improvement. Jaw thrust gives more than 50% improvement and lateral head rotation less than 50%. We therefore regard this as work in progress and presently prospectively reevaluate the effect of head rotation alone and head and trunk rotation. A subsequent study will include the use of a temporary OA that might mimic the effect of a definitive OA better than manual jaw thrust, while rotation of both head and trunk might be a better reflection of lateral sleep position than rotation of the head alone. We hope this will eventually lead to a good predictive model, which subsequently can be tested in prospective studies.

References

[1] Ferguson KA, Cartwright R, Rogers R, Schmidt-Nowara W. Oral appliances for snoring and obstructive sleep apnea: a review. Sleep. 2006; 29(2):244–262

[2] Johal A, Battagel JM, Kotecha BT. Sleep nasendoscopy: a diagnostic tool for predicting treatment success with mandibular advancement splints in obstructive sleep apnoea. Eur J Orthod. 2005; 27(6): 607–614

[3] Johal A, Hector MP, Battagel JM, Kotecha BT. Impact of sleep nasendoscopy on the outcome of mandibular advancement splint therapy in subjects with sleep-related breathing disorders. J Laryngol Otol. 2007; 121(7):668–675

[4] Vanderveken OM, Vroegop AV, Van de Heyning PH, Braem MJ. Drug-induced sleep endoscopy completed with a simulation bite approach for the prediction of the outcome of treatment of obstructive sleep apnea with mandibular repositioning appliances. Oper Tech Otolaryngol–Head Neck Surg. 2011; 22(2):175–182

[5] Vroegop AV, Vanderveken OM, Dieltjens M, et al. Sleep endoscopy with simulation bite for prediction of oral appliance treatment outcome. J Sleep Res. 2013; 22(3):348–355

[6] Benoist L, de Ruiter M, de Lange J, de Vries N. A randomized, controlled trial of positional therapy versus oral appliance therapy for position-dependent sleep apnea. Sleep Med. 2017; 34:109–117

[7] de Ruiter MHT, Benoist LBL, de Vries N, de Lange J. Durability of treatment effects of the Sleep Position Trainer versus oral appliance therapy in positional OSA: 12-month follow-up of a randomized controlled trial. Sleep Breath. 2017; 22(2):441–450

[8] Dieltjens M, Vroegop AV, Verbruggen AE, et al. A promising concept of combination therapy for positional obstructive sleep apnea. Sleep Breath. 2015; 19(2):637–644

[9] Vroegop AV, Vanderveken OM, Boudewyns AN, et al. Drug-induced sleep endoscopy in sleep-disordered breathing: report on 1,249 cases. Laryngoscope. 2014; 124(3):797–802

[10] Ravesloot MJ, de Vries N. One hundred consecutive patients undergoing drug-induced sleep endoscopy: results and evaluation. Laryngoscope. 2011; 121(12):2710–2716

[11] Vonk PE, Beelen AMEH, de Vries N. Towards a prediction model for drug-induced sleep endoscopy as selection tool for oral appliance treatment and positional therapy in obstructive sleep apnea. Sleep Breath. 2018; 22(4):901–907

[12] Cartwright RD. Effect of sleep position on sleep apnea severity. Sleep. 1984; 7(2):110–114

[13] Kim KT, Cho YW, Kim DE, Hwang SH, Song ML, Motamedi GK. Two subtypes of positional obstructive sleep apnea: Supine-predominant and supine-isolated. Clin Neurophysiol. 2016; 127(1):565–570

[14] Kezirian EJ, Hohenhorst W, de Vries N. Drug-induced sleep endoscopy: the VOTE classification. Eur Arch Otorhinolaryngol. 2011; 268 (8):1233–1236

[15] Koutsourelakis I, Safiruddin F, Ravesloot M, Zakynthinos S, de Vries N. Surgery for obstructive sleep apnea: sleep endoscopy determinants of outcome. Laryngoscope. 2012; 122(11):2587–2591

[16] Vanderveken OM, Maurer JT, Hohenhorst W, et al. Evaluation of drug-induced sleep endoscopy as a patient selection tool for implanted upper airway stimulation for obstructive sleep apnea. J Clin Sleep Med. 2013; 9(5):433–438

[17] Huntley C, Chou D, Doghramji K, Boon M. Preoperative Drug induced sleep endoscopy improves the surgical approach to treatment of

obstructive sleep apnea. Ann Otol Rhinol Laryngol. 2017; 126(6): 478–482

[18] Certal VF, Pratas R, Guimarães L, et al. Awake examination versus DISE for surgical decision making in patients with OSA: a systematic review. Laryngoscope. 2015

[19] Ravesloot MJL, White D, Heinzer R, Oksenberg A, Pépin JL. Efficacy of the new generation of devices for positional therapy for patients with positional obstructive sleep apnea: a systematic review of the literature and meta-analysis. J Clin Sleep Med. 2017; 13(6):813–824

[20] Hoekema A, Stegenga B, De Bont LG. Efficacy and co-morbidity of oral appliances in the treatment of obstructive sleep apnea-hypopnea: a systematic review. Crit Rev Oral Biol Med. 2004; 15(3):137–155

[21] van Kesteren ER, van Maanen JP, Hilgevoord AA, Laman DM, de Vries N. Quantitative effects of trunk and head position on the apnea hypopnea index in obstructive sleep apnea. Sleep (Basel). 2011; 34(8):1075–1081

[22] Zhu K, Bradley TD, Patel M, Alshaer H. Influence of head position on obstructive sleep apnea severity. Sleep Breath. 2017; 21(4):821–828

[23] Eichler C, Sommer JU, Stuck BA, Hörmann K, Maurer JT. Does drug-induced sleep endoscopy change the treatment concept of patients with snoring and obstructive sleep apnea? Sleep Breath. 2013; 17(1):63–68

[24] Safiruddin F, Koutsourelakis I, de Vries N. Analysis of the influence of head rotation during drug-induced sleep endoscopy in obstructive sleep apnea. Laryngoscope. 2014; 124(9):2195–2199

[25] Safiruddin F, Koutsourelakis I, de Vries N. Upper airway collapse during drug induced sleep endoscopy: head rotation in supine position compared with lateral head and trunk position. Eur Arch Otorhinolaryngol. 2015; 272(2):485–488

[26] Mador MJ, Kufel TJ, Magalang UJ, Rajesh SK, Watwe V, Grant BJ. Prevalence of positional sleep apnea in patients undergoing polysomnography. Chest. 2005; 128(4):2130–2137

[27] Oksenberg A. Positional and non-positional obstructive sleep apnea patients. Sleep Med. 2005; 6(4):377–378

[28] Richard W, Kox D, den Herder C, Laman M, van Tinteren H, de Vries N. The role of sleep position in obstructive sleep apnea syndrome. Eur Arch Otorhinolaryngol. 2006; 263(10):946–950

12 Complications of DISE

Ivor Kwame and Bhik Kotecha

Abstract

Drug-induced sleep endoscopy (DISE) is a safe and well-tolerated procedure. However, a constellation of patient, anesthetic and equipment factors may contribute to rare complications. In this chapter, some of the recognized complications of DISE are outlined and summarized in relation to excess airway secretions and/or apneic and hypopneic events. Several practical strategies to reduce the limited risks of DISE are discussed.

Keywords: obstructive sleep apnea, drug induced sleep endoscopy, complications

12.1 Introduction

We have already established in earlier chapters that fiberoptic nasal endoscopic (FNE) evaluation during drug-induced sleep endoscopy (DISE) is a method of investigating upper airways obstruction in patients with a spectrum of sleep-disordered breathing (SDB) conditions. DISE facilitates the real-time assessment of the dynamic airway changes during a pharmacological reproduction of the patients' own natural sleep.[1,2,3,4,5,6,7,8,9,10,11] This can aid informed decisions about suitably targeted therapy for components of the upper airways complex that are contributing most significantly to obstruction during the patient's natural sleep.[3,4,6,7,9,12]

DISE therefore necessitates the use of sedation without a secure airway. While this is not unique, the combination of the use of anesthetic agents in an often overweight, supine patient with an otherwise unprotected airway is peculiar to DISE and forms the source of potential risk. In this chapter, we explore some of the equipment, patient and anesthetic-related factors that potentially contribute to risk. Tips to mitigate against some of these will also be suggested.

12.2 Background

Flexible FNE is one of the commonest procedures carried out by otorhinolaryngologists. It provides real-time information about the anatomical idiosyncrasies of a patient's nasal cavity, larynx and pharynx. While it can be associated with some contact discomfort and occasional epistaxis, the procedure is generally well-tolerated among awake patients and is not linked with any particularly common side effects. FNE is often conducted among awake patients without local anesthesia.[13,14,15]

Sedation and general anesthesia are largely accepted as safe when conducted by an appropriately trained clinician in a properly monitored clinical environment[16] and are carried out many millions of time across the world each year, with the vast majority conducted without incident.[16,17]

While it is beyond the scope of this chapter to detail the full distinctions between sedation and general anesthesia, or indeed to give detailed recommendations about the preferred synergistic anesthetic combinations to produce optimal conditions for DISE, it is true to say that DISE is performed under deep sedation rather than full anesthesia and increasingly features the use of a variety of sedative agents; however, probably the commonest being propofol, a short-acting intravenous agent.[18,19] We will briefly discuss propofol later in the chapter.

The aim of sedation in DISE is to reduce alertness and mimic sleep. This is done by bringing patients to a reduced level of consciousness, such that the stimulation of FNE within the upper airway does not significantly disturb the patient's pharmacological sleeping state. Nonetheless, the marginal distinction between such reduced levels of consciousness and full anesthesia is that in DISE, every effort is made to avoid rendering the patient totally unarousable, that is, fully anesthetized. Many consider deep sedation and full general anesthesia to be part of the same spectrum.[16,17] However, full anesthesia tends to necessitate adjuncts to help protect the patient's airway, whereas with sedation, this is typically not required to the same degree, as the patient's own airway protective mechanisms are grossly intact, albeit reduced.[16,17,20]

To understand how combining a very safe, common, largely outpatient procedure such as FNE with the process of sedation can lead to complications, we will look at the individual components of risk in turn.

12.3 Complications

12.3.1 Equipment Factors

FNE is a routine assessment in many ENT consultations. In the awake patient, FNE may be conducted with or without the aid of decongestant local anesthesia.[13,14,15] This choice of anesthesia highlights the innately interactive nature of FNE assessment insomuch as whilst it is considered tolerable, patient feedback is utilized to determine how the nasal cavity is navigated. This interactivity between clinician and patient helps keep FNE tolerable in the awake patient. The lack of meaningful patient feedback during DISE means aggravation of the nasal lining is potentially more likely, with epistaxis and localized abrasion or ulceration being possible, although rarely seen.

FNE can also be linked with sneezing or sternutation, a forceful expulsion of air and upper airway secretions from the lungs via the nose and mouth.[21,22] It is a reflex reaction to perceived nasal irritation, whether chemical or physical, with afferent signals from the trigeminal nerve relayed to sneezing centers in the lateral medulla, resulting in efferent signals to the diaphragm, larynx, oral cavity and face.[22] An individual's threshold for sneezing is likely linked to genetic predisposition and can be observed with a range of stimuli whose mechanisms are not all clearly understood, including anesthetic agents, changes in room temperature, humidity or brightness.[21,22,23,24]

In the immediate aftermath of a sneeze, excess respiratory secretions and saliva can accumulate in and around the pharynx, bathing the larynx. These secretions are routinely swallowed in the awake patient, but as swallowing triggers are reduced in DISE, the secretions may accumulate in the supine patient and form an added threat to the airway due to laryngeal penetration, with risk of laryngospasm (which can induce pulmonary edema) or aspiration. It is noteworthy that anesthetic agents themselves can induce sneezing.[21,22,23]

12.3.2 Anesthetic Factors

It is beyond the scope of this chapter to detail recommended anesthetic regimes, and the precise anesthetic scope of complications will clearly relate to the specific combination of agents used during DISE. Nonetheless, as propofol is almost ubiquitously used in DISE, with or without the addition of other agents such as opioids or benzodiazepines, we will briefly discuss it here.

Propofol is useful in DISE, as it has rapid onset and is short-acting, meaning patients can be allowed to wake from the relatively quick assessment within a short period of time.[18,19] It is a nonopioid anesthetic agent with good amnesic but not analgesic effects, hence its frequent synergistic use with other agents.

Part of its mechanism of action through gamma–aminobutyric acid–A (GABA$_A$) and sodium channel receptors however is thought to induce spontaneous dysrhythmias as well as depress the respiratory system, by both reducing hypoxic drive and respiratory effort, encouraging apnea.[18,19] Some of the more common side effects of propofol use include pain at the injection site, especially when given in smaller veins, sneezing (as previously discussed), hypersalivation, reflux and hypotension, principally through systemic vasodilation and tissue fluid shifts. These are not necessarily unique to propofol alone.

There are several serious but rare complications of general anesthesia, beyond those already detailed with the direct use of propofol, which include seizures, dystonias, and impairment of renal and or liver function. Other drugs that are used during DISE include midazolam and dexmedetomidine, and it is important to bear

in mind the various adverse effects in relation to these drugs too.

12.3.3 Patient Factors

DISE is frequently performed in patients with known SDB. In this segment, we will first explore general patient factors to consider in DISE as well as those uniquely associated with SDB patients.

Patients may have predictable or idiosyncratic reactions to anesthetic agents, meaning they may respond to the agents by hypersalivating or producing excessive reflux during sedation. Sneezing is not uncommon during DISE and the threshold to sneeze is different for individual patients.[21,22,23,24] Excess secretions from hypersalivation, reflux, and/or sternutation, all add to the previously discussed airway threat.

While not all SDB patients are overweight, a significant proportion is.[25,26,27] Overweight patients are known to have increased anesthetic risks relating to their relatively narrowed oropharyngeal anatomy, which make timely tracheal intubation more difficult.[25,26,27,28,29] While intubation in DISE is rightly avoided, unexpected airway events may necessitate this being done in unfavorable conditions. Furthermore, excessive abdominal fat may reduce movement of the diaphragm on lying supine, leading to reduced tidal volumes and hypoxaemia.[27,28,29] These risks generally increase with increasing neck girth and obesity. Acid reflux is also commonly seen in overweight patients and the chronic perilaryngeal irritation may lower the threshold to laryngospasm.[30,31,32]

SDB patients with obstructive sleep apnea (OSA) by definition have frequent apneic episodes related to reduced hypoxic drive, and this is independent of their body habitus, but would add to the hypoxemia risk from a splinted diaphragm in obesity. Severe hypoxemia is particularly associated with cardiac ischemia and dysrhythmias.[18,19,26,28,29]

Other general patient risk factors in DISE relate to conditions not necessarily caused by but are commonly associated with SDB such as systemic hypertension, diabetes, renal impairment and pulmonary hypertension. These conditions have the potential of further complicating the sedation process.[28,29]

12.3.4 Recommendations

We have outlined that a range of complications may rarely arise during DISE in relation to inherent patient factors as well as factors that are equipment- and anesthesia-related. While some factors are unique to one domain or other, many factors crossover and are therefore compounded. These can be generally summarized under two broad areas of airway secretion and apnea-hypoxemia related. Whilst these factors may naturally occur in the patient during their own

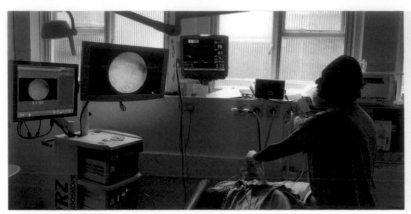

Fig. 12.1 Showing DISE performed on a screen next to anesthetic monitoring. Abbreviation: DISE, drug-induced sleep endoscopy.

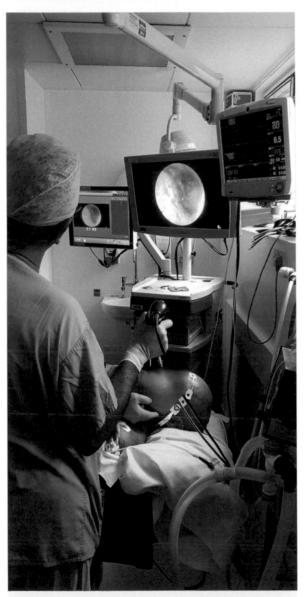

Fig. 12.2 Showing jaw thrust and use of BIS during DISE. Abbreviations: BIS, Bispectral index analysis; DISE, drug-induced sleep endoscopy.

physiological sleep, their hypoxic drive is further reduced during DISE; so, we would make the following practical recommendation:

- Excessive airway secretions: Avoid lying patient completely flat (e.g., use a pillow) and have low threshold for airway suctioning and/or antimuscarinics such as glycopyrrolate. Consider performing DISE on a screen, ideally near the anesthetic monitors (▶ Fig. 12.1), to encourage dual surgical and anesthetic awareness of airway/respiratory.
- Apneic-hypoxemia: Have a low threshold for use of airway maneuvers such as chin lift and jaw thrust during apnea (▶ Fig. 12.2), and consider having a preoperatively agreed nadir (e.g., 80% saturation) beyond which oxygen is given. Electroencephalography (EEG) monitoring such as bispectral index analysis (BIS) during DISE may also help in titrating anesthetic agents against sedation depth to further reduce the hypoxemia risk.[1]

These recommendations may dilute the pharmacological representation of the patient's own physiological sleep during DISE (e.g., instrumenting their pharynx during suctioning), but they also serve to dilute the scope of potential risks during DISE. The recommendations run alongside already well-known good perioperative care such as careful and appropriate preoperative planning and triage, as well as competent sedation in appropriately monitored clinical environment, with safe postprocedure observations.

12.4 Discussion

DISE remains a safe and well-tolerated procedure. However, a constellation of patient, anesthetic and equipment factors may contribute to rare complications. In this chapter, we have outlined some of the recognized complications of DISE and have summarized them in relation to excess airway secretions and/or apnea hypopnea. We have also outlined several practical strategies to further reduce the limited risks of DISE.

Our recommendations are not exhaustive and serve to run alongside appropriate perioperative anesthetic care, while appreciating that the need to avoid excessive intervention, which would further diverge the DISE process from the patient's own physiological sleep.

References

[1] Babar-Craig H, Rajani NK, Bailey P, Kotecha BT. Validation of sleep nasendoscopy for assessment of snoring with bispectral index monitoring. Eur Arch Otorhinolaryngol. 2012; 269(4):1277–1279

[2] Borowiecki B, Pollak CP, Weitzman ED, Rakoff S, Imperato J. Fibro-optic study of pharyngeal airway during sleep in patients with hypersomnia obstructive sleep-apnea syndrome. Laryngoscope. 1978; 88(8 Pt 1): 1310–1313

[3] Croft CB, Thomson HG, Samuels MP, Southall DP. Endoscopic evaluation and treatment of sleep-associated upper airway obstruction in infants and young children. Clin Otolaryngol Allied Sci. 1990; 15(3): 209–216

[4] De Vito A, Carrasco Llatas M, Vanni A, et al. European position paper on drug-induced sedation endoscopy (DISE). Sleep Breath. 2014; 18 (3):453–465

[5] Dijemeni E, Kotecha B. Drug-induced sedation endoscopy (DISE) DATA FUSION system: clinical feasibility study. Eur Arch Otorhinolaryngol. 2018; 275(1):247–260

[6] Hewitt RJ, Dasgupta A, Singh A, Dutta C, Kotecha BT. Is sleep nasendoscopy a valuable adjunct to clinical examination in the evaluation of upper airway obstruction? Eur Arch Otorhinolaryngol. 2009; 266(5): 691–697

[7] Kotecha B, De Vito A. Drug induced sleep endoscopy: its role in evaluation of the upper airway obstruction and patient selection for surgical and non-surgical treatment. J Thorac Dis. 2018; 10 Suppl 1: S40–S47

[8] Kotecha B, Kumar G, Sands R, Walden A, Gowers B. Evaluation of upper airway obstruction in snoring patients using digital video stroboscopy. Eur Arch Otorhinolaryngol. 2013; 270(7):2141–2147

[9] Kotecha BT, Hannan SA, Khalil HM, Georgalas C, Bailey P. Sleep nasendoscopy: a 10-year retrospective audit study. Eur Arch Otorhinolaryngol. 2007; 264(11):1361–1367

[10] Lechner M, Wilkins D, Kotecha B. A review on drug-induced sedation endoscopy: technique, grading systems and controversies. Sleep Med Rev. 2018; 41:141–148

[11] Pringle MB, Croft CB. A comparison of sleep nasendoscopy and the Müller manoeuvre. Clin Otolaryngol Allied Sci. 1991; 16(6):559–562

[12] Pringle MB, Croft CB. A grading system for patients with obstructive sleep apnoea-based on sleep nasendoscopy. Clin Otolaryngol Allied Sci. 1993; 18(6):480–484

[13] Sadek SA, De R, Scott A, White AP, Wilson PS, Carlin WV. The efficacy of topical anaesthesia in flexible nasendoscopy: a double-blind randomised controlled trial. Clin Otolaryngol Allied Sci. 2001; 26(1):25–28

[14] Lennox P, Hern J, Birchall M, Lund V. Local anaesthesia in flexible nasendoscopy. A comparison between cocaine and co-phenylcaine. J Laryngol Otol. 1996; 110(6):540–542

[15] Frosh AC, Jayaraj S, Porter G, Almeyda J. Is local anaesthesia actually beneficial in flexible fibreoptic nasendoscopy? Clin Otolaryngol Allied Sci. 1998; 23(3):259–262

[16] Vargo J, ed. Sedation and Monitoring in Gastrointestinal Endoscopy, An Issue of Gastrointestinal Endoscopy Clinics of North America. Philadelphia, Pennsylvania: Elsevier Health Sciences; 2016

[17] Vargo JJ, Niklewski PJ, Williams JL, Martin JF, Faigel DO. Patient safety during sedation by anesthesia professionals during routine upper endoscopy and colonoscopy: an analysis of 1.38 million procedures. Gastrointest Endosc. 2017; 85(1):101–108

[18] Bryson HM, Fulton BR, Faulds D. Propofol. An update of its use in anaesthesia and conscious sedation. Drugs. 1995; 50(3):513–559

[19] Symington L, Thakore S. A review of the use of propofol for procedural sedation in the emergency department. Emerg Med J. 2006; 23(2): 89–93

[20] Hillman DR, Platt PR, Eastwood PR. The upper airway during anaesthesia. Br J Anaesth. 2003; 91(1):31–39

[21] Ahn ES, Mills DM, Meyer DR, Stasior GO. Sneezing reflex associated with intravenous sedation and periocular anesthetic injection. Am J Ophthalmol. 2008; 146(1):31–35

[22] Virk JS, Kotecha B. Sneezing during drug-induced sedation endoscopy. Sleep Breath. 2014; 18(3):451–452

[23] Abramson DC. Sudden unexpected sneezing during the insertion of peribulbar block under propofol sedation. Can J Anaesth. 1995; 42 (8):740–743

[24] Semes LP, Amos JF, Waterbor JW. The photic sneeze response: a descriptive report of a clinic population. J Am Optom Assoc. 1995; 66 (6):372–377

[25] Dixon JB, Schachter LM, O'Brien PE, et al. Surgical vs conventional therapy for weight loss treatment of obstructive sleep apnea: a randomized controlled trial. JAMA. 2012; 308(11):1142–1149

[26] Foster GD, Borradaile KE, Sanders MH, et al. Sleep AHEAD Research Group of Look AHEAD Research Group. A randomized study on the effect of weight loss on obstructive sleep apnea among obese patients with type 2 diabetes: the Sleep AHEAD study. Arch Intern Med. 2009; 169(17):1619–1626

[27] Rubinstein I, Colapinto N, Rotstein LE, Brown IG, Hoffstein V. Improvement in upper airway function after weight loss in patients with obstructive sleep apnea. Am Rev Respir Dis. 1988; 138(5). 1192–1195

[28] Candiotti K, Sharma S, Shankar R. Obesity, obstructive sleep apnoea, and diabetes mellitus: anaesthetic implications. Br J Anaesth. 2009; 103 Suppl 1:i23–i30

[29] Siyam M, Benhamou D, eds. Anaesthetic management of adult patients with obstructive sleep apnea syndrome. Ann Fr Anesth Reanim. 2007;26(1):39–52

[30] Toohill RJ. Role of refluxed acid in pathogenesis of laryngeal disorders. Am J Med. 1997; 103 5A:100S–106S

[31] Maceri DR, Zim S. Laryngospasm: an atypical manifestation of severe gastroesophageal reflux disease (GERD). Laryngoscope. 2001; 111(11 Pt 1):1976–1979

[32] Loughlin CJ, Koufman JA. Paroxysmal laryngospasm secondary to gastroesophageal reflux. Laryngoscope. 1996; 106(12 Pt 1):1502–1505

13 DISE and Treatment Outcome

Anneclaire V.M.T. Vroegop, Olivier M. Vanderveken, Ioannis Koutsourelakis, Madeline J.L. Ravesloot, and Nico de Vries

Abstract

Drug-induced sleep endoscopy (DISE) has predictive value in patient selection for upper airway (UA) surgery and UA stimulation. In this chapter, the following specific modalities will be discussed: pharyngeal surgery, hypoglossal nerve stimulation, transoral robotic surgery (TORS), positional therapy, and surgical failures. It can also be of value in selecting patients for mandibular advancement device (MAD) treatment.

Keywords: obstructive sleep apnea, drug induced sleep endoscopy, treatment outcome

13.1 Introduction

Drug-induced sleep endoscopy (DISE) has an additional value in optimizing patient selection for surgical upper airway (UA) interventions and can also be helpful in selecting patients for mandibular advancement device (MAD) treatment.[1,2,3,4,5] Nonetheless, the association between DISE findings and surgical outcome are still subject of further research to consolidate the role of DISE in patient selection.[6] For this purpose, several perioperative maneuvers were introduced, as described in Chapter 11. It was demonstrated that DISE has a relevant influence on recommendations for treatment location when compared to awake assessment, including endoscopic examination. This is particularly true when considering MAD treatment or tongue base interventions and difference in hypopharyngeal or laryngeal obstruction; however, it has also been mentioned that high-quality evidence level studies with statistically appropriate sample sizes and clinical cross-validations are necessary to further determine the role of DISE in the assessment of treatment outcomes.[7,8,9,10,11]

13.2 Predictive Value

DISE could modify surgical treatment options and procedures in 50% of obstructive sleep apnea (OSA) patients, but the available published studies lack evidence on the association between this impact and surgical outcomes.[11] However, patient selection based on site-specific upper airway (UA) behavior has proved to be of value in improving treatment outcome.[6,12,13,14,15,16,17,18]

More specifically, a complete circular collapse of the palate can be associated with less favorable surgical outcomes for UA simulation therapy, although a recent report showed similar improvement in patients with isolated retropalatal collapse as compared to other types of collapse with regard to apnea–hypopnea index (AHI).[14,19]

In a study assessing the predictive value of DISE variables in patients undergoing UA surgery, it was found that in 49 patients undergoing UA surgery (palatal surgery, and/or radiofrequency ablation of the tongue base, and/or hyoid suspension) after DISE, nonresponders (53%) had a higher occurrence of complete or partial circumferential collapse at velum and complete anteroposterior collapse at tongue base or epiglottis in comparison with responders; the presence of complete circumferential collapse at velum and of complete anteroposterior collapse at tongue base were the only independent predictors of UA surgery failure.[6]

In a report on 34 patients (body mass index [BMI] 34.4 kg/m^2) who underwent DISE and UA surgery, Soares et al found an overall surgical success rate of 56% and a greater incidence of severe lateral oropharyngeal wall collapse (73.3 vs. 36.8%) and severe supraglottic collapse (93.3 vs. 63.2%) in the surgical failure group as compared to the surgical success group.[17] When discussing the role of the lateral wall, the prominence and restriction due to thickening of the lateral pharyngeal wall and increased parapharyngeal fat volume have to be taken into account.[20]

A recent multicenter study showed surgical response was associated with tonsil size and BMI (inversely), and oropharyngeal lateral wall-related obstruction was also associated with poorer surgical outcomes, as complete tongue-related obstruction was associated with a lower odds of surgical response in moderate to severe OSA; surgical outcomes were not clearly associated with the degree and configuration of velum-related obstruction or the degree of epiglottis-related obstruction.[21]

It must be mentioned that comparison of a variety of study results from different sleep centers across the world is challenging, as standardization for DISE is lacking.[22]

13.3 Treatment Outcome Per Modality

In this section, the results of studies with a focus on the role of DISE in patient selection for a (site-)specific procedure are discussed.

13.3.1 Pharyngeal Surgery

As for the treatment of snoring, patient selection for uvulopalatopharyngoplasty (UPPP) or soft palate laser surgery tended to improve if guided by DISE, based on the identification of velar vibration/obstruction.[23,24]

Oropharyngeal surgery in isolated soft palate obstruction leads to an subjective improvement of 69% and AHI reduction to below 15/hour sleep in a study of Hessel et al.[2]

Based on site of obstruction during DISE, Iwanaga et al found that the post-UPPP improvement rate was 74.4% for soft palatal type of obstruction, 76.2% for the tonsillar type, 53.3% for the circumferential palatal type, and 34.0% for the mixed type, concluding that treatment produced excellent or good effects for the soft palatal and tonsillar types of obstruction, and many patients with the circumferential palatal and mixed types of obstruction showed only some improvement or no change.[25]

A study on expansion sphincter pharyngoplasty (ESP) showed that palatal circumferential narrowing and bulky lateral pharyngeal tissue are favorable surgical indications for ESP in patients with OSA, with a significant reduction in mean AHI from 35.5 to 17.3/hour sleep postoperatively.[13] In a cohort of patients with AHI values ranging from 5 to 70/hour sleep and a lateral collapse of the oropharynx during DISE, Plaza et al found that ESP as a standalone treatment has a reasonable chance of being successful with minimal morbidity.

As for barbed reposition pharyngoplasty (BRP) as a standalone procedure or as part of a multilevel approach, patients with a main site of obstruction at the retropalatal level, with or without retrolingual obstruction, can also be expected to have reasonable outcomes in terms of success and minimal morbidity.[26]

13.3.2 Hypoglossal Nerve Therapy

Vanderveken et al found a significantly better outcome with UA stimulation (UAS) therapy in patients without palatal complete concentric collapse (CCC), reducing AHI from 37.6/hour sleep to 11.1/hour sleep, without statistical difference noted in AHI or BMI at baseline between the patients with and without palatal CCC.[19]

A recent study of Mahmoud et al showed post-UAS AHI to be 5.7/hour sleep for patients with isolated retropalatal collapse and 3.9/hour sleep for other patients ($p = 0.888$), postoperative nadir oxyhemoglobin saturation (NOS) was 92% among patients with isolated retropalatal collapse, and 91% for others ($p = 0.402$), concluding that patients with isolated retropalatal collapse showed similar improvement to other types of collapse with regard to AHI and NOS.[14]

13.3.3 Transoral Robotic Surgery

Transoral robotic surgery (TORS) appears to be a promising and safe procedure for patients, seeking an alternative to traditional therapy, with appropriate patient selection remaining important for successful implementation and requiring further research.[27] Meraj et al reported on 100 patients who underwent TORS and multilevel procedures, leading to improvement of AHI in 87 patients, but based on DISE findings, no predictive patterns for treatment success could be identified; however, patients with lateral oropharyngeal collapse were suggested to be poorer candidates.[28]

13.3.4 Maxillomandibular Advancement (MMA)

The role of DISE for patient selection for maxillomandibular advancement (MMA) surgery has been described, with AHI and oxygen desaturation index (ODI) improvement after MMA being best correlated with increased lateral pharyngeal wall stability, based on VOTE scoring.[29,30]

13.3.5 Positional Therapy

As for patients with positional obstructive sleep apnea syndrome (OSAS), it has been reported in literature that head rotation improves UA collapse during DISE in supine position, and this improvement of UA patency is more predominant in positional obstructive sleep apnea (POSA) patients.[31] A study of Victores et al demonstrated nearly all patients with POSA (91%) had at least a partial improvement in collapse while in the lateral sleep position, with most of this reduction involving the tongue base and epiglottis, whereas sleep position did not significantly alter the UA morphology of patients with nonpositional OSA.[32] DISE in multiple sleep positions should thus be considered as part of a minimally invasive approach to surgical therapy of OSA.

13.4 DISE in Surgical Failures

DISE may enhance the understanding of mechanisms leading to residual UA obstruction and could in some cases explain surgical failure, but the occurrence of clinically less relevant obstruction site(s) has also been reported.[33,34] In a cross-sectional study of DISE findings among 33 nonresponders (AHI 43.4 −/+ 26.6/hour sleep) to previous pharyngeal surgery, the majority of patients showed residual palatal obstruction, and almost all demonstrated hypopharyngeal obstruction; in addition, moderate-to-severe mouth opening occurred in one-third of subjects and was associated with narrowing of UA dimensions, concluding that residual UA obstruction in surgery nonresponders likely occurs due to multiple mechanisms.[34]

References

[1] Johal A, Hector MP, Battagel JM, Kotecha BT. Impact of sleep nasendoscopy on the outcome of mandibular advancement splint therapy in subjects with sleep-related breathing disorders. J Laryngol Otol. 2007; 121(7):668–675

[2] Hessel NS, de Vries N. Results of uvulopalatopharyngoplasty after diagnostic workup with polysomnography and sleep endoscopy: a report of 136 snoring patients. Eur Arch Otorhinolaryngol. 2003; 260 (2):91–95

[3] Vanderveken OM. Drug-induced sleep endoscopy (DISE) for non-CPAP treatment selection in patients with sleep-disordered breathing. Sleep Breath. 2013; 17(1):13–14

[4] Battagel JM, Johal A, Kotecha BT. Sleep nasendoscopy as a predictor of treatment success in snorers using mandibular advancement splints. J Laryngol Otol. 2005; 119(2):106–112

[5] Johal A, Battagel JM, Kotecha BT. Sleep nasendoscopy: a diagnostic tool for predicting treatment success with mandibular advancement splints in obstructive sleep apnoea. Eur J Orthod. 2005; 27(6):607–614

[6] Koutsourelakis I, Safiruddin F, Ravesloot M, Zakynthinos S, de Vries N. Surgery for obstructive sleep apnea: sleep endoscopy determinants of outcome. Laryngoscope. 2012; 122(11):2587–2591

[7] Eichler C, Sommer JU, Stuck BA, Hörmann K, Maurer JT. Does drug-induced sleep endoscopy change the treatment concept of patients with snoring and obstructive sleep apnea? Sleep Breath. 2013; 17(1):63–68

[8] Campanini A, Canzi P, De Vito A, Dallan I, Montevecchi F, Vicini C. Awake versus sleep endoscopy: personal experience in 250 OSAHS patients. Acta Otorhinolaryngol Ital. 2010; 30(2):73–77

[9] Gillespie MB, Reddy RP, White DR, Discolo CM, Overdyk FJ, Nguyen SA. A trial of drug-induced sleep endoscopy in the surgical management of sleep-disordered breathing. Laryngoscope. 2013; 123(1):277–282

[10] Hewitt RJ, Dasgupta A, Singh A, Dutta C, Kotecha BT. Is sleep nasendoscopy a valuable adjunct to clinical examination in the evaluation of upper airway obstruction? Eur Arch Otorhinolaryngol. 2009; 266(5): 691–697

[11] Certal VF, Pratas R, Guimarães L, et al. Awake examination versus DISE for surgical decision making in patients with OSA: A systematic review. Laryngoscope. 2016; 126(3):768–774

[12] Plaza G, Baptista P, O'Connor-Reina C, Bosco G, Pérez-Martín N, Pang KP. Prospective multi-center study on expansion sphincter pharyngoplasty. Acta Otolaryngol. 2019; 139(2):219–222

[13] Hong SN, Kim HG, Han SY, et al. Indications for and outcomes of expansion sphincter pharyngoplasty to treat lateral pharyngeal collapse in patients with obstructive sleep apnea. JAMA Otolaryngol Head Neck Surg. 2019; 145(5):405–412

[14] Mahmoud AF, Thaler ER. Outcomes of hypoglossal nerve upper airway stimulation among patients with isolated retropalatal collapse. Otolaryngol Head Neck Surg. 2019; 160(6):1124–1129

[15] Wang Y, Sun C, Cui X, Guo Y, Wang Q, Liang H. The role of drug-induced sleep endoscopy: predicting and guiding upper airway surgery for adult OSA patients. Sleep Breath. 2018; 22(4):925–931

[16] Hsu YS, Jacobowitz O. Does sleep endoscopy staging pattern correlate with outcome of advanced palatopharyngoplasty for moderate to severe obstructive sleep apnea? J Clin Sleep Med. 2017; 13(10):1137–1144

[17] Soares D, Sinawe H, Folbe AJ, et al. Lateral oropharyngeal wall and supraglottic airway collapse associated with failure in sleep apnea surgery. Laryngoscope. 2012; 122(2):473–479

[18] Blumen M, Bequignon E, Chabolle F. Drug-induced sleep endoscopy: a new gold standard for evaluating OSAS? Part II: Results. Eur Ann Otorhinolaryngol Head Neck Dis. 2017; 134(2):109–115

[19] Vanderveken OM, Maurer JT, Hohenhorst W, et al. Evaluation of drug-induced sleep endoscopy as a patient selection tool for implanted upper airway stimulation for obstructive sleep apnea. J Clin Sleep Med. 2013; 9(5):433–438

[20] Schwab RJ, Gupta KB, Gefter WB, Metzger LJ, Hoffman EA, Pack AI. Upper airway and soft tissue anatomy in normal subjects and patients with sleep-disordered breathing. Significance of the lateral pharyngeal walls. Am J Respir Crit Care Med. 1995; 152(5 Pt 1): 1673–1689

[21] Green KK, Kent DT, D'Agostino MA, et al. Drug-induced sleep endoscopy and surgical outcomes: a multicenter cohort study. Laryngoscope. 2019; 129(3):761–770

[22] Chong KB, De Vito A, Vicini C. Drug-induced sleep endoscopy in treatment options selection. Sleep Med Clin. 2019; 14(1):33–40

[23] Camilleri AE, Ramamurthy L, Jones PH. Sleep nasendoscopy: what benefit to the management of snorers? J Laryngol Otol. 1995; 109 (12):1163–1165

[24] El Badawey MR, McKee G, Heggie N, Marshall H, Wilson JA. Predictive value of sleep nasendoscopy in the management of habitual snorers. Ann Otol Rhinol Laryngol. 2003; 112(1):40–44

[25] Iwanaga K, Hasegawa K, Shibata N, et al. Endoscopic examination of obstructive sleep apnea patients during drug-induced sleep. Acta Otolaryngol Suppl. 2003(550):36–40

[26] Montevecchi F, Meccariello G, Firinu E, et al. Prospective multicentre study on barbed reposition pharyngoplasty standing alone or as a part of multilevel surgery for sleep apnoea. Clin Otolaryngol. 2018; 43(2):483–488

[27] Vicini C, Montevecchi F, Gobbi R, De Vito A, Meccariello G. Transoral robotic surgery for obstructive sleep apnea syndrome: Principles and technique. World J Otorhinolaryngol Head Neck Surg. 2017; 3(2): 97–100

[28] Meraj TS, Muenz DG, Glazer TA, Harvey RS, Spector ME, Hoff PT. Does drug-induced sleep endoscopy predict surgical success in transoral robotic multilevel surgery in obstructive sleep apnea? Laryngoscope. 2017; 127(4):971–976

[29] Liu SY, Huon LK, Iwasaki T, et al. Efficacy of maxillomandibular advancement examined with drug-induced sleep endoscopy and computational fluid dynamics airflow modeling. Otolaryngol Head Neck Surg. 2016; 154(1):189–195

[30] Kezirian EJ, Hohenhorst W, de Vries N. Drug-induced sleep endoscopy: the VOTE classification. Eur Arch Otorhinolaryngol. 2011; 268 (8):1233–1236

[31] Safiruddin F, Koutsourelakis I, de Vries N. Analysis of the influence of head rotation during drug-induced sleep endoscopy in obstructive sleep apnea. Laryngoscope. 2014; 124(9):2195–2199

[32] Victores AJ, Hamblin J, Gilbert J, Switzer C, Takashima M. Usefulness of sleep endoscopy in predicting positional obstructive sleep apnea. Otolaryngol Head Neck Surg. 2014; 150(3):487–493

[33] Blumen MB, Latournerie V, Bequignon E, Guillere L, Chabolle F. Are the obstruction sites visualized on drug-induced sleep endoscopy reliable? Sleep Breath. 2015; 19(3):1021–1026

[34] Kezirian EJ. Nonresponders to pharyngeal surgery for obstructive sleep apnea: insights from drug-induced sleep endoscopy. Laryngoscope. 2011; 121(6):1320–1326

14 DISE and Position-Dependent OSA

Madeline J.L. Ravesloot, Patty E. Vonk, and Nico de Vries

Abstract

In the majority of patients with obstructive sleep apnea (OSA), the frequency and duration of apneas are influenced by body position, most often the supine position. A crucial aspect in positional (PP) is that severity of disease is completely dependent on the time spent in the supine posture; thus, avoiding the supine position through positional therapy can be a valuable therapeutic option.

Historically, drug-induced sleep endoscopy (DISE) is performed in the supine position. Various studies have found significantly different findings in OSA patients when comparing findings in supine position versus nonsupine position. In PP, it is recommended to perform DISE in both the lateral body position as well as the supine position.

Keywords: sleep apnea, obstructive/therapy, supine position, positional therapy, compliance, positional, obstructive sleep apnea, body position

14.1 Positional Sleep Apnea

In approximately 56 to 75% of patients with obstructive sleep apnea (OSA), the frequency and duration of apneas are influenced by body position.[1,2,3,4,5,6] Various definitions of position-dependent obstructive sleep apnea (POSA) have been applied in the literature. The most common classification system and definition used today makes a distinction between two groups: positional (PP)[7] and nonpositional OSA (NPP).[3,4,8] In PP, desaturations, cyclic variations in heart rate, loud snoring, and apneas/hypopneas appear almost exclusively in the supine position (▶ Fig. 14.1).[9] Cartwright first described the arbitrary cutoff point of a difference of 50% or more in apnea index between supine and nonsupine positions.[3] In the medical literature, modified versions have been introduced, adding cutoff values for the overall apnea-hypopnea index (AHI), AHI in supine and nonsupine position, and time spent in the various sleeping positions.[8,10,11,12]

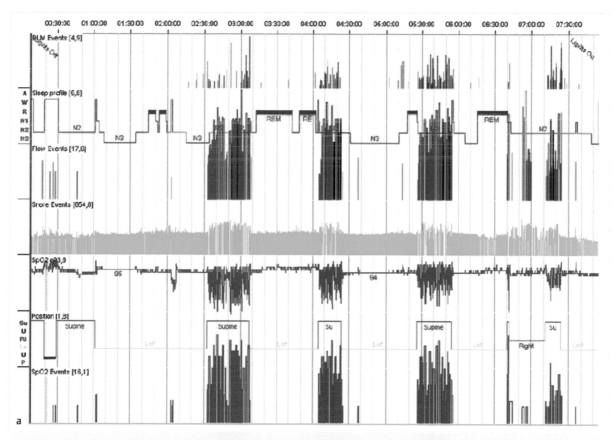

Fig. 14.1 (a) The positional (PP) obstructive sleep apnea (OSA) patient: desaturations, cyclic variations in heart rate, loud snoring, and apneas/hypopneas appear almost exclusively in the supine position.

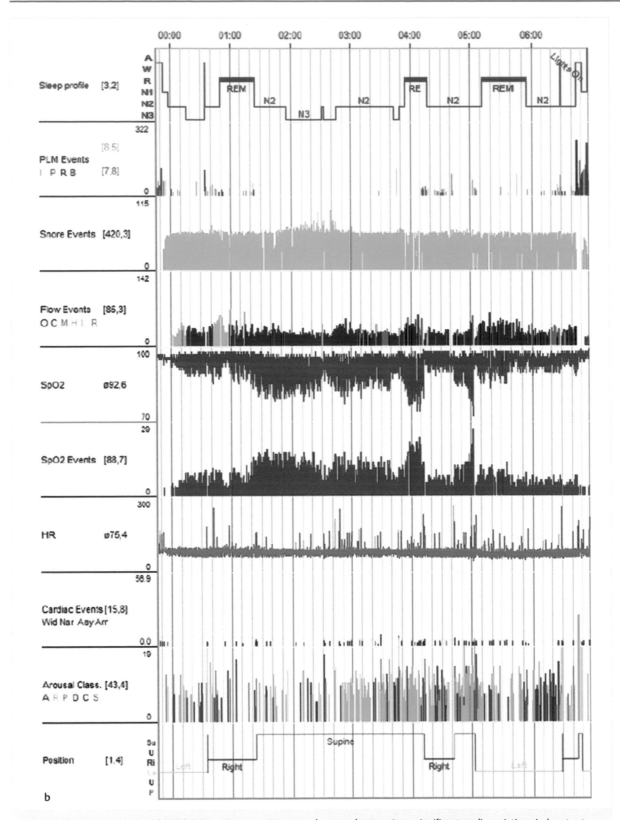

Fig. 14.1 (b) The non-positional (NPP) OSA patient: continuous and severe desaturations, significant cyclic variations in heart rate, constant and loud snoring, and a high number of apneas/hypopneas appear independent of body position.

The prevalence of POSA decreases as the severity of sleep apnea increases. The majority of POSA patients (70–80%) are afflicted with it in its mild or moderate form.[2,4,5,12] Furthermore, POSA patients in comparison with NPP have a lower body mass index (BMI) and are younger.[2,4,5,13] The prevalence of POSA is thought to be higher in Asian populations.[14,15,16]

14.2 Management of POSA

A crucial aspect in PP is that severity of disease is completely dependent on the time spent in the supine posture. Bearing this in mind, avoidance of the supine position is a valuable therapeutic option.

Positional therapy (PT) is aimed at preventing patients from sleeping in the worst sleeping position (WSP).[2] In most cases, sleeping supine is the WSP.[2,17] Various techniques have been described, but the majority of studies on PT use the so-called tennis ball technique (TBT): a bulky mass strapped to the patient's back.[1] Even though TBT is simple and cheap, as well as effective in reducing the AHI, results are unsatisfactory. Backache, discomfort and no improvement, or even a deterioration of sleep quality or daytime alertness, have been responsible for poor compliance and subsequent disappointing long-term results.[1,18] Compliance rates reported in the literature range from 40 to 70% in the short-term to only 10% in the long-term.[1,19,20,21]

Recent developments have seen the introduction of a new generation of small, lightweight, battery-powered devices for PT, which apply vibrotactile feedback.[1,10,22,23] These small devices are either attached to the neck (e.g., Night Shift: Advanced BrainMonitoring, Inc., Carlsbad, CA, USA) or chest (e.g., Night Balance Lunoa and Sleep Position Trainer, Koninklijke Philips N.V., The Netherlands) with a strap. When the supine position is identified, the device provides a vibrating stimulus to cause the patient to turn to a nonsupine sleeping position.[24] These devices are simple to use for patients and clinicians and are reversible.

There is strong evidence that the new devices for PT are effective in reducing the AHI during short-term follow-up.[25] In a recent meta-analysis, when combining data for studies reporting on the effect of PT, there was a mean difference (MD) of 11.3/hour (54% reduction) and 33.6% (84% reduction) in AHI and in percentage total sleeping time (TST) in the supine position. The standardized mean difference for both parameters demonstrated a large magnitude of effect (> 0.8 in both cases).[25] Several studies also found improvements in excessive daytime sleepiness and quality of life as measured using various questionnaires (e.g., Epworth sleepiness scale, ESS; functional outcome of sleep questionnaire, FOSQ).[24,25]

When interpreting results of conservative treatment approaches, it is important to take into consideration that the effectiveness of a treatment reducing respiratory indices depends not only on the effect on upper airway (UA) obstruction, but also on compliance.[7,26,27]

Under short-term study conditions (1 month), follow-up median compliance of new generation PT devices is high, varying from 76 to 96%, when defined as 4 hours/night, 7 nights/week.[7,23,28] Data on long-term follow-up is limited, but similar to other conservative treatment modalities for OSA, where one recognizes a bimodal distribution (50% discontinuation rate).[24,26,29,30,31] Patients either tolerate the device well or not at all. Although self-evident, poor early compliance predicts poor long-term compliance.[32]

Reported long-term (6–12 months) compliance in patients who continue using the device is high, ranging from 75 to 82%, when defined as 4 hours/night, 7 nights/week.[30,31] Median hours of use per night ranged from 5.2 to 5.5 hours.[29,31]

Suitable candidates for PT are those who will benefit from a clinically significant improvement of their OSA with the therapy, bearing in mind that patients could benefit from a combination of therapies.[33]

Description of patients who will or will not benefit from this mode of therapy have been explored.[34] In a recent paper describing the Amsterdam positional OSA classification (APOC) criteria, three categories were defined[35]:

1. *The true PP* has a nonsupine AHI < 5 events/hour. By avoiding the supine position, the patient can theoretically be cured.
2. *The NPP patient* who will not benefit from PT since his or her breathing abnormalities during sleep are not influenced by sleeping position.
3. *The multifactorial patient, who can benefit from PT but not be cured.* The multifactorial patient's OSA severity is influenced, in part, by sleep position.
   - Patients with a nonsupine AHI in a lower OSA severity category than the overall AHI. If treated with PT, the patient can theoretically decrease overall AHI and OSA severity category. As a consequence, patients can be treated with less aggressive primary treatment (e.g., less invasive surgery).
   - In patients who do not tolerate continuous positive airway pressure (CPAP) or oral appliances, PT can be considered as salvage therapy. For example, as the AHI drops, so does the CPAP pressure needed, potentially improving adherence.

Various nomenclatures have been described in the literature for patients whose respiratory disturbances normalize in the nonsupine position such as the true positional patient, POSA exclusive (ePOSA), supine-isolated OSA (siOSA) and APOC 1.[33,36,37,38]

Studies report a prevalence of 26 to 38% in OSA patients and 36 to 54% in POSA, with a prevalence decreasing with

OSA severity.[2,6,12] Translating these findings into clinical practice, a third of OSA patients could be ideal candidates for PT.

When considering PT as a treatment modality, there are a few further considerations:

- Studies suggest that through wearing polysomnography (PSG) apparatus, patients are likely to spend more time in the supine position (approximately 33%) than during normal sleep. Therefore, in both clinical practice and research, one must keep into consideration that PSG apparatus leads to an increase in percentage of total time spent in supine position and subsequently influences OSA severity measured by PSG, especially in PP (REF Heisenberg Vonk et al., HNO).[10,39,40,41,42]
- It is hypothesized that patients self-correct. Studies suggest an inverse relationship between the supine AHI and the TST% in supine position. Patients with the most severe disease while supine tend to avoid this position during sleep.[33,43]
- Obviously, patients unable to sleep in the lateral position due to shoulder problems or other disabilities are not good candidates for PT.[33]
- PT may not suffice for POSA patients who snore in all body positions and seek treatment for their snoring complaints.
- Besides POSA patients, PT is a treatment option for patients without sleep apnea, but snore solely in the supine position.[44] Although less relevant for the scope of this book, other patient groups include patients with position-dependent mixed or central apnea or pregnant women afflicted with POSA.[45]

14.3 Characteristics of Patients with POSA

Various studies using a variety of diagnostic modalities in awake patients have suggested that PP in comparison to NPP have more backward positioning of the lower jaw, lower facial height, longer posterior airway space (PAS) measurements, and smaller volume of lateral pharyngeal wall tissue and therefore greater lateral diameter and ellipsoid shape of the UA.[46,47,48,49,50] Also, PP tend to have a smaller neck circumference.[12] The current hypothesis is that even though the anterior–posterior[15] diameter in both PP and NPP is reduced as a result of the effect of gravity in the supine position, due to the greater lateral diameter in PP, there is sufficient preservation of airway space and avoidance of complete UA collapse. Furthermore, it has been suggested that a fall in functional residual lung capacity when moving from lateral to supine position may be an important triggering factor in the occurrence of POSA.[51]

Studies demonstrate the head position, separate from trunk position, as an important parameter to measure in patients with POSA.[52,53] Van Kesteren et al concluded that in a quarter of all OSA patients, the head position is an important additional factor next to the position of the trunk.[51] In these patients, the AHI calculated whilst the head is in a supine position is higher than the AHI determined over the time when the trunk is in supine position. Furthermore, 6.5% of patients were not position-dependent, based on the position sensor on the trunk, and were classified as only head supine dependent. This finding may have consequences for diagnosis and treatment of OSA patients in the future.

14.4 DISE and POSA

DISE is not a prerequisite when prescribing PT, but when performing DISE in PP, certain considerations are of importance.

Historically, DISE is performed in the supine position (▶ Fig. 14.2a). Although it may be technically easier to perform the procedure in the supine position, various studies have found significantly different DISE findings in supine

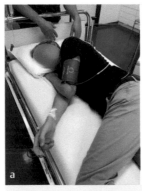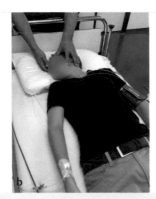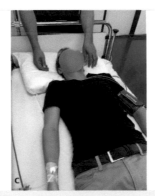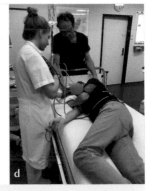

Fig. 14.2 Positioning of the patient during drug-induced sleep endoscopy (DISE). **(a)** Head and trunk in the lateral position. **(b)** Head in lateral position, trunk in supine position. **(c)** Head and trunk in supine position. **(d)** DISE in lateral head and trunk position.

position versus nonsupine position. Lee et al found statistically significant improvement in the following anatomical structures, contributing to airway obstruction when the body position was changed from supine to lateral: soft palate, tongue base and larynx.[54] Prevalence of lateral wall obstruction was not affected by position change. However, persistent obstruction at the level of the lateral walls in the nonsupine position in NPP was more frequent in comparison to PP. In a small-scale study by Victores et al, the majority of patients with POSA (91%) had, at least, a partial improvement in collapse, while in the lateral sleep position in comparison to the supine position. Most of the reduction involved the tongue base and epiglottis. In NPP, the author's demonstrated that sleep position did not significantly alter the UA morphology.[55]

Vonk et al described the phenomenon that a primary epiglottic collapse, not secondary to tongue base collapse (e.g., floppy epiglottis), was solely present in supine position and to a lesser extent when the head was rotated during DISE. They did not find the presence of a floppy epiglottis when patients were positioned in laterally.[56]

Although it may be technically easier to perform DISE in the supine position (► Fig. 14.2a), one must bear in mind that the majority of OSA patients are positional and have an increase in respiratory events, specifically in the supine question; therefore, it goes without saying that one should examine an individual's pattern of UA obstruction in both the lateral and supine position.

Studies have questioned whether rotation of the head to the lateral position (► Fig. 14.2b) may suffice instead of positioning of the head and trunk in the lateral position (► Fig. 14.2c). In NPP, findings concerning UA patency during DISE are similar when comparing lateral head rotation and lateral head and trunk rotation.[56] However, in PP, this is not the case.

In PP, it is recommended to perform DISE in both the lateral body position (► Fig. 14.2c) as well as the supine position (► Fig. 14.2a). From experience, we recommend starting the DISE with the patient positioned on the right side, both head and trunk (► Fig. 14.2d). After adequate observation in this position, tilt the patient into the supine position (both head and trunk).

14.5 Surgery and POSA

DISE is used for surgical treatment planning.

After UA surgery for OSA, studies report that 42 to 75% of NPP improve to less severe PP.[58,59,60,61,62,63,64,65] The effect of surgery is suggested to be greater in the lateral position than supine position, resulting in residual OSA in the supine position. Concerning preoperative PP, 50 to 90% remain positional.[59,60,62] Studies report the beneficial effects of adjuvant PT in patients with postoperative persistent POSA.[63,65,66]

It remains unclear whether position dependency is a predictor for surgical success. Various small-scale studies evaluating different surgical modalities report on this matter. No difference was found in surgical success rate between NPP and PP undergoing uvulopalatopharyngoplasty (UPPP),[59] isolated tongue base or multilevel surgery,[60] and UA stimulation.[68] Other studies suggest that position dependency is a prognostic factor for surgical success, Li et al found that PP undergoing relocation pharyngoplasty had a greater chance of surgical success.[62] Other studies were in favor of NPP: Lee et al reported that patients who failed UPPP were predominantly positional;[68] van Maanen et al found that NPP who underwent UPPP or zetapalatopharyngoplasty (ZPP) and radiofrequency of the base of tongue had a greater chance of surgical success in comparison to PP;[63] and Kastoer et al found a lower efficacy of UA surgery in PP as compared to NPP.[64]

There is a significant clinical diversity in these studies, complicating the interpretation of the results, such as different forms of UA surgery and different definitions of surgical success and POSA. Not only is the level of evidence poor but studies are also generally small-scale and retrospective. Another important consideration is that the inverse relationship of BMI and AHI is not only related to PP but also to surgical success. Considering these confounders is of the utmost importance. Finally, a consideration that cannot be ignored is that the severity of POSA is strongly dependent on the time spent in supine position.

References

[1] Ravesloot MJ, van Maanen JP, Dun L, de Vries N. The undervalued potential of positional therapy in position-dependent snoring and obstructive sleep apnea-a review of the literature. Sleep Breath. 2013; 17(1):39–49

[2] Ravesloot MJ, Frank MH, van Maanen JP, Verhagen EA, de Lange J, de Vries N. Positional OSA part 2: retrospective cohort analysis with a new classification system (APOC). Sleep Breath. 2016; 20(2):881–888

[3] Cartwright RD. Effect of sleep position on sleep apnea severity. Sleep. 1984; 7(2):110–114

[4] Oksenberg A, Silverberg DS, Arons E, Radwan H. Positional vs nonpositional obstructive sleep apnea patients: anthropomorphic, nocturnal polysomnographic, and multiple sleep latency test data. Chest. 1997; 112(3):629–639

[5] Richard W, Kox D, den Herder C, et al. The role of sleep position in obstructive sleep apnea syndrome. European archives of oto-rhino-laryngology: official journal of the European Federation of Oto-Rhino-Laryngological Societies (EUFOS): affiliated with the German Society for Oto-Rhino-Laryngology. Head Neck Surg. 2006; 263:946–950

[6] Heinzer R, Petitpierre NJ, Marti-Soler H, Haba-Rubio, J. Prevalence and characteristics of positional sleep apnea in the HypnoLaus population-based cohort. Sleep Med. 2018; 48–157–162

[7] Eijsvogel MM, Ubbink R, Dekker J, et al. Sleep position trainer versus tennis ball technique in positional obstructive sleep apnea syndrome. J Clin Sleep Med. 2015; 11(2):139–147

[8] Marklund M, Persson M, Franklin KA. Treatment success with a mandibular advancement device is related to supine-dependent sleep apnea. Chest. 1998; 114(6):1630–1635

[9] Oksenberg A, Gadoth N. Are we missing a simple treatment for most adult sleep apnea patients? The avoidance of the supine sleep position. J Sleep Res. 2014; 23(2):204–210

[10] Bignold JJ, Mercer JD, Antic NA, McEvoy RD, Catcheside PG. Accurate position monitoring and improved supine-dependent obstructive sleep apnea with a new position recording and supine avoidance device. J Clin Sleep Med. 2011; 7(4):376–383

[11] Permut I, Diaz-Abad M, Chatila W, et al. Comparison of positional therapy to CPAP in patients with positional obstructive sleep apnea. J Clin Sleep Med. 2010; 6(3):238–243

[12] Mador MJ, Kufel TJ, Magalang UJ, Rajesh SK, Watwe V, Grant BJ. Prevalence of positional sleep apnea in patients undergoing polysomnography. Chest. 2005; 128(4):2130–2137

[13] Itasaka Y, Miyazaki S, Ishikawa K, Togawa K. The influence of sleep position and obesity on sleep apnea. Psychiatry Clin Neurosci. 2000; 54(3):340–341

[14] Mo JH, Lee CH, Rhee CS, Yoon IY, Kim JW. Positional dependency in Asian patients with obstructive sleep apnea and its implication for hypertension. Arch Otolaryngol Head Neck Surg. 2011; 137(8): 786–790

[15] Teerapraipruk B, Chirakalwasan N, Simon R, et al. Clinical and polysomnographic data of positional sleep apnea and its predictors. Sleep Breath. 2012; 16(4):1167–1172

[16] Tanaka F, Nakano H, Sudo, N, Kubo, C. Relationship between the body position-specific apnea–hypopnea index and subjective sleepiness. Respiration. 2009; 78(2):185:90

[17] Cartwright RD, Diaz F, Lloyd S. The effects of sleep posture and sleep stage on apnea frequency. Sleep. 1991; 14(4):351–353

[18] Ravesloot MJ, Benoist L, van Maanen P, et al. Novel positional devices for the treatment of positional obstructive sleep apnea, and how this relates to sleep surgery. Adv Otorhinolaryngol. 2017;80:28–36

[19] Bignold JJ, Deans-Costi G, Goldsworthy MR, et al. Poor long-term patient compliance with the tennis ball technique for treating positional obstructive sleep apnea. J Clin Sleep Med. 2009; 5(5):428–430

[20] Oksenberg A, Silverberg D, Offenbach D, Arons E. Positional therapy for obstructive sleep apnea patients: A 6-month follow-up study. Laryngoscope. 2006; 116(11):1995–2000

[21] Heinzer RC, Pellaton C, Rey V, et al. Positional therapy for obstructive sleep apnea: an objective measurement of patients' usage and efficacy at home. Sleep Med. 2012; 13(4):425–428

[22] van Maanen JP, Richard W, Van Kesteren ER, et al. Evaluation of a new simple treatment for positional sleep apnoea patients. J Sleep Res. 2012; 21(3):322–329

[23] Levendowski DJ, Seagraves S, Popovic D, Westbrook PR. Assessment of a neck-based treatment and monitoring device for positional obstructive sleep apnea. J Clin Sleep Med. 2014; 10(8):863–871

[24] Vonk P, Ravesloot M. Positional obstructive sleep apnea. Somnologie (Berl). 2018; 22:79–84

[25] Ravesloot MJL, White D, Heinzer R, Oksenberg A, Pépin JL. Efficacy of the new generation of devices for positional therapy for patients with positional obstructive sleep apnea: a systematic review of the literature and meta-analysis. J Clin Sleep Med. 2017; 13(6):813–824

[26] Ravesloot MJ, de Vries N. Reliable calculation of the efficacy of nonsurgical and surgical treatment of obstructive sleep apnea revisited. Sleep (Basel). 2011; 34(1):105–110

[27] Ravesloot MJ, de Vries N, Stuck BA. Treatment adherence should be taken into account when reporting treatment outcomes in obstructive sleep apnea. Laryngoscope. 2014; 124(1):344–345

[28] van Maanen JP, Meester KA, Dun LN, et al. The sleep position trainer: a new treatment for positional obstructive sleep apnoea. Sleep Breath. 2013; 17(2):771–779

[29] van Maanen JP, de Vries N. Long-term effectiveness and compliance of positional therapy with the sleep position trainer in the treatment of positional obstructive sleep apnea syndrome. Sleep (Basel). 2014; 37(7):1209–1215

[30] Laub RR, Tønnesen P, Jennum PJ. A sleep position trainer for positional sleep apnea: a randomized, controlled trial. J Sleep Res. 2017; 26 (5):641–650

[31] de Ruiter MHT, Benoist LBL, de Vries N, de Lange J. Durability of treatment effects of the Sleep Position Trainer versus oral appliance therapy in positional OSA: 12-month follow-up of a randomized controlled trial. Sleep Breath. 2018; 22(2):441–450

[32] Levendowski D, Cunnington D, Swieca J, Westbrook P. User compliance and behavioral adaptation associated with supine avoidance therapy. Behav Sleep Med. 2018; 16(1):27–37

[33] Gadoth NOA. Positional therapy in obstructive sleep apnea: for whom and for whom not. In: de Vries N, Ravesloot MJL, van Maanen JP, eds. Positional Therapy in Obstructive Sleep Apnea. New York: Springer; 2015:383–394

[34] Oksenberg A, Silverberg DS. The effect of body posture on sleep-related breathing disorders: facts and therapeutic implications. Sleep Med Rev. 1998; 2(3):139–162

[35] Frank MH, Ravesloot MJ, van Maanen JP, Verhagen E, de Lange J, de Vries N. Positional OSA part 1: Towards a clinical classification system for position-dependent obstructive sleep apnoea. Sleep Breath. 2015; 19(2):473–480

[36] Kim KT, Cho YW, Kim DE, Hwang SH, Song ML, Motamedi GK. Two subtypes of positional obstructive sleep apnea: Supine-predominant and supine-isolated. Clin Neurophysiol. 2016; 127(1):565–570

[37] Joosten SA, Edwards BA, Wellman A, et al. The Effect of body position on physiological factors that contribute to obstructive sleep apnea. Sleep (Basel). 2015; 38(9):1469–1478

[38] Heinzer R, Vat S, Marques-Vidal P, et al. Prevalence of sleep-disordered breathing in the general population: the HypnoLaus study. Lancet Respir Med. 2015; 3(4):310–318

[39] Metersky ML, Castriotta RJ. The effect of polysomnography on sleep position: possible implications on the diagnosis of positional obstructive sleep apnea. Respiration. 1996; 63(5):283–287

[40] Wimaleswaran H, Yo S, Buzacott H, et al. Sleeping position during laboratory polysomnography compared to habitual sleeping position at home. Journal of Sleep Research. 2018; 27(S2):e40_12766

[41] Logan MB, Branham GH, Eisenbeis JF, et al. 11:48 am: unattended home monitoring in the evaluation of sleep apnea: is it equal to formal polysomnograph? Otolaryngol Head Neck Surg. 1996; 115:156–P56

[42] Vonk PE, de Vries N, Ravesloot MJL. Polysomnography and sleep position: a Heisenberg phenomenon? HNO 2019 Sep;67(9):679–684

[43] Kaur A, Verma R, Gandhi A, et al. 0631 Effect of disease severity on determining body position during sleep in patients with positional obstructive sleep apnea. Journal of Sleep and Sleep Disorders Research. 2017; 40:A233–A33

[44] Benoist LBL, Beelen AMEH, Torensma B, de Vries N. Subjective effects of the sleep position trainer on snoring outcomes in position-dependent non-apneic snorers. Eur Arch Otorhinolaryngol. 2018; 275(8):2169–2176

[45] Morong S, Hermsen B, de Vries N. Sleep-disordered breathing in pregnancy: a review of the physiology and potential role for positional therapy. Sleep Breath. 2014; 18(1):31–37

[46] Saigusa H, Suzuki M, Higurashi N, Kodera K. Three-dimensional morphological analyses of positional dependence in patients with obstructive sleep apnea syndrome. Anesthesiology. 2009; 110(4): 885–890

[47] Chang ET, Shiao GM. Craniofacial abnormalities in Chinese patients with obstructive and positional sleep apnea. Sleep Med. 2008; 9(4): 403–410

[48] Walsh JH, Leigh MS, Paduch A, et al. Effect of body posture on pharyngeal shape and size in adults with and without obstructive sleep apnea. Sleep. 2008; 31(11):1543–1549

[49] Soga T, Nakata S, Yasuma F, et al. Upper airway morphology in patients with obstructive sleep apnea syndrome: effects of lateral positioning. Auris Nasus Larynx. 2009; 36(3):305–309

[50] Pevernagie DA, Stanson AW, Sheedy PF, II, Daniels BK, Shepard JW, Jr. Effects of body position on the upper airway of patients with obstructive sleep apnea. Am J Respir Crit Care Med. 1995; 152(1): 179–185

[51] Joosten SA, Sands SA, Edwards BA, et al. Evaluation of the role of lung volume and airway size and shape in supine-predominant obstructive sleep apnoea patients. Respirology. 2015; 20(5):819–827

[52] van Kesteren ER, van Maanen JP, Hilgevoord AA, Laman DM, de Vries N. Quantitative effects of trunk and head position on the apnea hypopnea index in obstructive sleep apnea. Sleep (Basel). 2011; 34(8): 1075–1081

[53] Zhu K, Bradley TD, Patel M, Alshaer H. Influence of head position on obstructive sleep apnea severity. Sleep Breath. 2017; 21(4):821–828

[54] Lee CH, Kim DK, Kim SY, Rhee CS, Won TB. Changes in site of obstruction in obstructive sleep apnea patients according to sleep position: a DISE study. Laryngoscope. 2015; 125(1):248–254

[55] Victores AJ, Hamblin J, Gilbert J, Switzer C, Takashima M. Usefulness of sleep endoscopy in predicting positional obstructive sleep apnea. Otolaryngol Head Neck Surg. 2014; 150(3):487–493

[56] Vonk PE, Ravesloot MJL, Kasius KM, van Maanen JP, de Vries N. Floppy epiglottis during drug-induced sleep endoscopy: an almost complete resolution by adopting the lateral posture. Sleep Breath. 2020; 24(1):103–109

[57] Vonk PE, van de Beek MJ, Ravesloot MJL, de Vries N. Drug-induced sleep endoscopy: new insights in lateral head rotation compared to lateral head and trunk rotation in (non)positional obstructive sleep apnea patients. Laryngoscope. 2019; 129(10):2430–2435

[58] Katsantonis GP, Miyazaki S, Walsh JK. Effects of uvulopalatopharyngoplasty on sleep architecture and patterns of obstructed breathing. Laryngoscope. 1990; 100(10 Pt 1):1068–1072

[59] Lee CH, Kim S-W, Han K, et al. Effect of uvulopalatopharyngoplasty on positional dependency in obstructive sleep apnea. Arch Otolaryngol Head Neck Surg. 2011; 137(7):675–679

[60] van Maanen JP, Ravesloot MJ, Witte BI, Grijseels M, de Vries N. Exploration of the relationship between sleep position and isolated tongue base or multilevel surgery in obstructive sleep apnea. Eur Arch Otorhinolaryngol. 2012; 269(9):2129–2136

[61] Lee YC, Eun YG, Shin SY, Kim SW. Change in position dependency in non-responders after multilevel surgery for obstructive sleep apnea:

analysis of polysomnographic parameters. Eur Arch Otorhinolaryngol. 2014; 271(5):1081–1085

[62] Li H-Y, Cheng W-N, Chuang L-P, et al. Positional dependency and surgical success of relocation pharyngoplasty among patients with severe obstructive sleep apnea. Otolaryngol Head Neck Surg. 2013; 149(3):506–512

[63] van Maanen JP, Witte BI, de Vries N. Theoretical approach towards increasing effectiveness of palatal surgery in obstructive sleep apnea: role for concomitant positional therapy? Sleep Breath. 2014; 18(2):341–349

[64] Kastoer C, Benoist LBL, Dieltjens M, et al. Comparison of upper airway collapse patterns and its clinical significance: drug-induced sleep endoscopy in patients without obstructive sleep apnea, positional and non-positional obstructive sleep apnea. Sleep Breath. 2018; 22(4):939–948

[65] Benoist LB, de Ruiter MH, de Lange J, et al. Residual POSA after maxillomandibular advancement in patients with severe OSA. In: de Vries, N, Ravesloot MJL, van Maanen PM. Positional Therapy in Obstructive Sleep Apnea: New York: Springer; 2015:321–329

[66] Benoist LBL, Verhagen M, Torensma B, van Maanen JP, de Vries N. Positional therapy in patients with residual positional obstructive sleep apnea after upper airway surgery. Sleep Breath. 2017; 21(2):279–288

[67] Steffen A, Hartmann JT, König IR, Ravesloot MJL, Hofauer B, Heiser C. Evaluation of body position in upper airway stimulation for obstructive sleep apnea-is continuous voltage sufficient enough? Sleep Breath. 2018; 22(4):1207–1212

[68] Lee CH, Shin H-W, Han DH, et al. The implication of sleep position in the evaluation of surgical outcomes in obstructive sleep apnea. Otolaryngol Head Neck Surg. 2009; 140(4):531–535

15 Significance of Complete Concentric Collapse of the Palate

Eli Van de Perck and Olivier M. Vanderveken

Abstract

Complete concentric collapse of the palate is the result of both anteroposterior (AP) and lateral narrowing of the velopharyngeal wall. Its prevalence during DISE is 10 to 31.5%. Several studies have demonstrated a clear relationship with a high body mass index (BMI), and most of them have also shown a positive correlation with the severity of obstructive sleep apnea (OSA). DISE remains the mainstay of its diagnosis; it is an important diagnostic finding with multiple therapeutic implications.

Keywords: obstructive sleep apnea, drug induced sleep endoscopy, complete concentric collapse

15.1 Introduction

Complete concentric collapse of the palate (CCCp) is the result of both anteroposterior (AP) and lateral narrowing of the velopharyngeal wall. This endoscopic feature can be readily distinguished from AP collapse of the palate by its funnel-shaped, sphincter-like appearance (▶ Fig. 15.1). The prevalence of CCCp during drug-induced sleep endoscopy (DISE) ranges from 10 to 31.5%.[1,2,3,4,5] Several studies have demonstrated a clear relationship between CCCp and a high body mass index (BMI),[2,3,4,5,6] and most of them have also shown a positive correlation with the severity of obstructive sleep apnea (OSA) in terms of apnea–hypopnea index (AHI).[2,3,4] Nevertheless, DISE remains the mainstay of diagnosis of CCCp, since anthropometric and sleep measurements alone are not accurate enough to predict this pathophysiological condition, which is also referred to as a specific DISE phenotype in patients with OSA.[4] The presence of CCCp is an important diagnostic finding with multiple therapeutic implications.[1,7,8]

15.2 Pathophysiology: Upper Airway Shape and Collapsibility

The importance of upper airway (UA) shape in the pathogenesis of OSA was first recognized by Leiter in 1996.[9] He compared two UA shapes—both ellipses, one with the long axis oriented in the AP dimension, and one with the long axis oriented in the lateral dimension— and postulated that the former shape predisposes to OSA. He reckoned that muscles along the lateral walls are inactive during apneic events, and dilating UA muscles primarily stabilize or expand the UA in the AP dimension. Consequently, the mechanical effectiveness of the dilating muscles depends on the accompanying UA shape; muscle activity increases the UA area to a lesser extent in the AP-shaped ellipse than in the lateral equivalent. This hypothesis was in agreement with previous clinical evidence of increased lateral narrowing with concentric-to-elliptical UA configurations in apneic subjects compared to healthy controls during awake magnetic resonance imaging (MRI).[10,11] Ciscar and colleagues later on confirmed these findings during natural sleep.[12] In their study with ultrafast MRI, subjects with OSA generally showed smaller concentric shapes of the velopharynx, as compared to healthy controls who generally showed larger elliptical shapes with the long axis oriented in the lateral dimension.

A recent study concerning the influence of collapse patterns during DISE on continuous positive airway pressure (CPAP) levels has demonstrated a positive correlation between CCCp (together with partial concentric collapse) and CPAP levels (mean pressure 9.19 cmH$_2$O *vs.* 7.21 cmH$_2$O).[13] Therapeutic CPAP levels are considered predictive for UA collapsibility, with high-pressure levels corresponding to

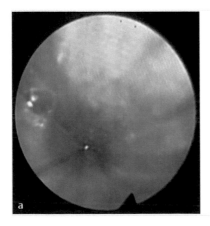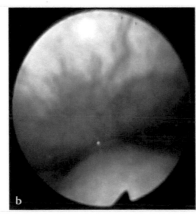

Fig. 15.1 Complete concentric **(a)** *versus* complete AP **(b)** collapse at the level of the palate during DISE. Abbreviations: AP, anteroposterior; DISE, drug-induced sleep endoscopy.

more positive pharyngeal critical closing pressures (Pcrit), and vice versa.[14] Taken together, CCCp during DISE might be a marker of increased UA collapsibility in OSA patients.

The clear relationship between CCCp and BMI might be explained by adipose tissue deposition in the pharynx. Koenig and Thach studied the effects of mass loading on UA shape and collapsibility using an animal model.[15] They positioned loads on the anterior neck region of anesthetized rabbits in order to simulate accumulation of adipose tissue. Mass loading caused a concentric narrowing of the velo- and oropharynx during endoscopy, and decreased the stability of the UA, leading to an increased (*i.e.,* less negative) closing pressure.

In summary, CCCp might reflect decreased UA stability, as a result of increased extraluminal tissue pressure related to cervical fat accumulation on the one hand,[16] and ineffective compensatory activity of the pharyngeal musculature on the other hand. Nevertheless, the current evidence on this subject is sparse and requires further investigation.

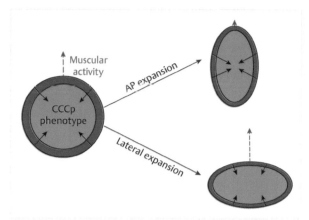

Fig. 15.2 The effect of AP and lateral expansion of the UA on CCCp. Abbreviations: AP, anteroposterior; CCCp, complete concentric collapse of the palate; UA, upper airway.

15.3 Predictive Value on Treatment Outcome

15.3.1 Pharyngeal Surgery

The presence of CCCp has been formerly associated to an increased risk of treatment failure after pharyngeal surgery.[1,17] Palatal surgery consisted, in these studies, generally of conventional uvulopalatopharyngoplasty (UPPP). Conforming to the hypothesis of Leiter (Chapter 17.2), this type of surgery might worsen the UA shape in cases of concentric narrowing by nullifying the mechanical benefit of the dilating pharyngeal muscles, and approximating the lateral walls (► Fig. 15.2). Consequently, several surgical techniques have been introduced with the primary aim of UA expansion in the lateral dimension.[18,19,20] Studies based on these techniques have demonstrated favorable reductions in AHI in patients with the CCCp phenotype during DISE.[21,22,23] Moreover, according to Hasselbacher and colleagues, pharyngeal surgery with lateral expansion might effectively eliminate CCCp.[24] They evaluated the effects of modified UPPP surgery on UA collapse patterns in 15 CPAP-intolerant patients with previous diagnosis of CCCp. Three months after surgery, only one patient showed persistent CCCp during follow-up DISE, while one patient showed no residual collapse of the palate, and 13 patients showed AP collapse of the palate (of which nine were partial and four complete). These results indicate that pharyngeal surgery might open the door for upper airway stimulation (UAS) treatment in patients who are initially excluded due to the presence of CCCp.

Anteroposterior expansion reduces the mechanical benefit of the pharyngeal musculature and pulls the lateral walls in, leading to an unchanged, or even increased, UA

instability. Lateral expansion, on the other hand, produces a synergistic effect by ameliorating the effectiveness of the pharyngeal musculature in maintaining UA patency.

15.3.2 Upper Airway Stimulation (UAS)

A prospective feasibility study in 2012 identified CCCp for the first time as a negative predictive factor for UAS, using electrical neurostimulation of the hypoglossal nerve.[25] Seven subjects underwent DISE before implantation and all four subjects with CCCp appeared to be nonresponders. Consecutive validation of CCCp as an exclusion criterion (together with BMI ≥32 kg/m[2] and AHI > 50 events/hour) for UAS revealed a significant reduction in AHI among treated patients. Vanderveken and colleagues subsequently confirmed the negative predictive value of CCCp for UAS outcome in a larger cohort of 21 patients with OSA.[7] This time, five patients presented with CCCp, and all of them failed to achieve a significant reduction in AHI six months after UAS implantation (mean baseline AHI 41.5 events/hour *vs.* AHI with UAS 48.1 events/hour). The remaining patients with AP collapse of the palate, however, demonstrated a significant improvement (mean baseline AHI 37.6 events/hour *vs.* AHI with UAS 11.6 events/hour). Based on these findings, CCCp was considered a formal exclusion criterion in the large pivotal cohort study evaluating UAS for OSA, known as the STAR trial,[26] which led to the Food and Drug Administration (FDA) approval of UAS treatment for selected patients with OSA. Since the absence of CCCp during DISE is often regarded as the strictest eligibility criterion, no other data is available on UAS in patients with CCCp.

The presence of isolated AP collapse of the palate, on the other hand, can be effectively treated by UAS, showing no differences with other forms of UA collapse.[27] One possible explanation for retropalatal opening during stimulation of the hypoglossal nerve is the so-called palatoglossal coupling.[28] This mechanical linkage between the palate and tongue body produces an anterior and inferior displacement of the palate during tongue protrusion and might lead to a multilevel effect of hypoglossal nerve stimulation.

15.3.3 Mandibular Advancement Device Treatment

The negative predictive value of CCCp for mandibular advancement device (MAD) treatment was recently demonstrated in a prospective study of 100 patients with OSA.[8] Together with complete lateral oropharyngeal collapse, CCCp significantly increased the odds of treatment deterioration, defined as an increase in AHI with MAD compared to the baseline AHI. These results suggest that MAD expands the UA in a similar longitudinal fashion as UAS.[29] As such, UAS and MAD can be optimal treatments for patients with AP collapse patterns, and suboptimal for patients with concentric collapse patterns.

15.3.4 Maxillomandibular Advancement Surgery

Kastoer and colleagues recently assessed the association between UA collapse patterns and the outcome after maxillomandibular advancement (MMA) surgery in a cohort of 19 patients with OSA.[30] As a result, they found an equal AHI reduction in patients with and without CCCp. Furthermore, all six patients who were previously diagnosed with CCCp showed a conversion to AP collapse (4/6) or complete resolution of the collapse (2/6) at the level of the palate during postoperative DISE. The authors concluded that CCCp does not influence treatment outcome after MMA, and CCCp can be effectively eliminated by this kind of surgery.

15.4 Summary

CCCp is regarded as a distinct feature during DISE in patients with OSA. This specific DISE phenotype probably results from simultaneous AP and lateral narrowing of the velopharyngeal wall and corresponds to an increased collapsibility of the UA.

Evidence in the literature clearly indicates that OSA patients with CCCp should be excluded from therapy with UAS and/or mandibular advancement device MAD, as a high probability of nonresponse and failure can be anticipated. MMA outcomes are not related to the presence of CCCp, and MMA seems to be able to eliminate CCCp. Patients with CCCp can become proper candidates for UAS and/or MAD treatment when postoperative DISE evaluation after MMA or specific pharyngeal surgery confirms the elimination of this specific DISE phenotype.

References

[1] Koutsourelakis I, Safiruddin F, Ravesloot M, Zakynthinos S, de Vries N. Surgery for obstructive sleep apnea: sleep endoscopy determinants of outcome. Laryngoscope. 2012; 122(11):2587–2591

[2] Ravesloot MJ, de Vries N. One hundred consecutive patients undergoing drug-induced sleep endoscopy: results and evaluation. Laryngoscope. 2011; 121(12):2710–2716

[3] Vroegop AV, Vanderveken OM, Boudewyns AN, et al. Drug-induced sleep endoscopy in sleep-disordered breathing: report on 1,249 cases. Laryngoscope. 2014; 124(3):797–802

[4] Steffen A, Frenzel H, Wollenberg B, König IR. Patient selection for upper airway stimulation: is concentric collapse in sleep endoscopy predictable? Sleep Breath. 2015; 19(4):1373–1376

[5] Ong AA, Murphey AW, Nguyen SA, et al. Efficacy of upper airway stimulation on collapse patterns observed during drug-induced sedation endoscopy. Otolaryngol Head Neck Surg. 2016; 154(5):970–977

[6] Lan MC, Liu SY, Lan MY, Modi R, Capasso R. Lateral pharyngeal wall collapse associated with hypoxemia in obstructive sleep apnea. Laryngoscope. 2015; 125(10):2408–2412

[7] Vanderveken OM, Maurer JT, Hohenhorst W, et al. Evaluation of drug-induced sleep endoscopy as a patient selection tool for implanted upper airway stimulation for obstructive sleep apnea. J Clin Sleep Med. 2013; 9(5):433–438

[8] Op de Beeck S, Dieltjens M, Verbruggen AE, et al. Phenotypic labeling using drug-induced sleep endoscopy improves patient selection for mandibular advancement device outcome. J Clin Sleep Med. 2019; 15 (8 Epub ahead of print)

[9] Leiter JC. Upper airway shape: is it important in the pathogenesis of obstructive sleep apnea? Am J Respir Crit Care Med. 1996; 153(3): 894–898

[10] Rodenstein DO, Dooms G, Thomas Y, et al. Pharyngeal shape and dimensions in healthy subjects, snorers, and patients with obstructive sleep apnoea. Thorax. 1990; 45(10):722–727

[11] Schwab RJ, Gupta KB, Gefter WB, Metzger LJ, Hoffman EA, Pack AI. Upper airway and soft tissue anatomy in normal subjects and patients with sleep-disordered breathing. Significance of the lateral pharyngeal walls. Am J Respir Crit Care Med. 1995; 152(5 Pt 1): 1673–1689

[12] Ciscar MA, Juan G, Martínez V, et al. Magnetic resonance imaging of the pharynx in OSA patients and healthy subjects. Eur Respir J. 2001; 17(1):79–86

[13] Lan MC, Hsu YB, Lan MY, et al. The predictive value of drug-induced sleep endoscopy for CPAP titration in OSA patients. Sleep Breath. 2018; 22(4):949–954

[14] Landry SA, Joosten SA, Eckert DJ, et al. Therapeutic CPAP level predicts upper airway collapsibility in patients with obstructive sleep apnea. Sleep (Basel). 2017; 40(6)

[15] Koenig JS, Thach BT. Effects of mass loading on the upper airway. J Appl Physiol (1985). 1988; 64(6):2294–2299

[16] Kairaitis K, Howitt L, Wheatley JR, Amis TC. Mass loading of the upper airway extraluminal tissue space in rabbits: effects on tissue pressure and pharyngeal airway lumen geometry. J Appl Physiol (1985). 2009; 106(3):887–892

[17] Iwanaga K, Hasegawa K, Shibata N, et al. Endoscopic examination of obstructive sleep apnea syndrome patients during drug-induced sleep. Acta Otolaryngol Suppl. 2003(550):36–40

[18] Cahali MB, Formigoni GG, Gebrim EM, Miziara ID. Lateral pharyngoplasty versus uvulopalatopharyngoplasty: a clinical, polysomnographic and computed tomography measurement comparison. Sleep. 2004; 27(5):942–950

[19] Pang KP, Woodson BT. Expansion sphincter pharyngoplasty: a new technique for the treatment of obstructive sleep apnea. Otolaryngol Head Neck Surg. 2007; 137(1):110–114

[20] Vicini C, Hendawy E, Campanini A, et al. Barbed reposition pharyngo-plasty (BRP) for OSAHS: a feasibility, safety, efficacy and teachability pilot study. "We are on the giant's shoulders". Eur Arch Otorhinolar-yngol. 2015; 272(10):3065–3070

[21] Hsu YS, Jacobowitz O. Does sleep endoscopy staging pattern correlate with outcome of advanced palatopharyngoplasty for moderate to severe obstructive sleep apnea? J Clin Sleep Med. 2017; 13(10):1137–1144

[22] Hong SN, Kim HG, Han SY, et al. Indications for and outcomes of expansion sphincter pharyngoplasty to treat lateral pharyngeal col-lapse in patients with obstructive sleep apnea. JAMA Otolaryngol Head Neck Surg. 2019; 145(5):405–412

[23] Mantovani M, Carioli D, Torretta S, Rinaldi V, Ibba T, Pignataro L. Barbed snore surgery for concentric collapse at the velum: The Alianza technique. J Craniomaxillofac Surg. 2017; 45(11):1794–1800

[24] Hasselbacher K, Seitz A, Abrams N, Wollenberg B, Steffen A. Complete concentric collapse at the soft palate in sleep endoscopy: what change is possible after UPPP in patients with CPAP failure? Sleep Breath. 2018; 22(4):933–938

[25] Van de Heyning PH, Badr MS, Baskin JZ, et al. Implanted upper airway stimulation device for obstructive sleep apnea. Laryngoscope. 2012; 122(7):1626–1633

[26] Strollo PJ, Jr, Soose RJ, Maurer JT, et al. STAR Trial Group. Upper-airway stimulation for obstructive sleep apnea. N Engl J Med. 2014; 370(2):139–149

[27] Mahmoud AF, Thaler ER. Outcomes of hypoglossal nerve upper airway stimulation among patients with isolated retropalatal collapse. Otolaryngol Head Neck Surg. 2019; 160(6):1124–1129

[28] Heiser C, Edenharter G, Bas M, Wirth M, Hofauer B. Palatoglossus coupling in selective upper airway stimulation. Laryngoscope. 2017; 127(10):E378–E383

[29] Safiruddin F, Vanderveken OM, de Vries N, et al. Effect of upper-airway stimulation for obstructive sleep apnoea on airway dimensions. Eur Respir J. 2015; 45(1):129–138

[30] Kastoer C, Op de Beeck S, Dom M, et al. Drug-induced sleep endoscopy upper airway collapse patterns and maxillomandibular advancement. Laryngoscope. 2019

16 Epiglottic Collapse

Patty E. Vonk, Madeline J.L. Ravesloot, and Nico de Vries

Abstract

Most sleep surgeons are traditionally most uncomfortable about what to do in case of the finding of an epiglottic collapse (EC) during drug-induced sleep endoscopy (DISE). There is much controversy and uneasiness about what to do in such a case. The data discussed in this chapter indicate that EC appears almost exclusively in supine body position and to a lesser extent during lateral head (and trunk) rotation.

Keywords: obstructive sleep apnea, drug induced sleep endoscopy, positional obstructive sleep apnea

16.1 Introduction

Of the four levels of the VOTE classification system—velum, oropharynx, tongue base and epiglottis[1]—most sleep surgeons are traditionally most uncomfortable about what to do in case of the finding of an epiglottic collapse (EC) during drug-induced sleep endoscopy (DISE). While for the other three levels of the collapsible part of the upper airway (UA), many established surgical procedures are widely accepted and commonly performed (velum: palatal procedures; oropharynx: tonsillectomy and tonsillotomy; tongue base: upper airway stimulation [UAS], radio frequent ablation, hyoid suspension, genioglossal advancement, midline glossectomy, etc.), there is much more controversy and uneasiness about what to do in case of an EC.

Many definitions of an EC are applied in literature, resulting in a wide variation of the prevalence of an EC ranging from 9.7 to 73.5%.[2] First, an EC can be secondary to an anteroposterior (AP) collapse of the tongue base, pushing the epiglottis backward (▸ Fig. 16.1a, b). Second, a lateral collapse can originate from, for example, an underdevelopment of the epiglottis itself. Third, an EC can be isolated moving from AP, which is also called a floppy epiglottis (FE) or trapdoor phenomenon (▸ Fig. 16.2). Most ECs are AP, while the lateral, pediatric type of obstruction occurs less often. In this chapter, we will focus on the phenomenon of an isolated EC, since treatment approach, specifically UA surgery, will differ between the two.

Treatment, either conservative or surgical, of an isolated EC can be challenging. First, a FE has been linked to continuous positive airway pressure (CPAP) failure, suggesting that, in certain cases, the epiglottis is pushed further backward on application of CPAP.[3,4,5] (In case of suspicion of CPAP failure due to a FE, DISE can be performed during CPAP usage). Furthermore, previous studies have shown that treatment with a mandibular advancement device (MAD) for this type of collapse can be difficult and is often not successful.[3,4,5,6] To predict whether MAD treatment will be successful, DISE can be performed to see if an isolated EC can be resolved by applying jaw thrust. In case of a positive reaction, it is felt, but not proven, that treatment with a MAD would make sense. It has to be realized that this is based on expert opinion, but evidence in the literature on this topic is lacking.

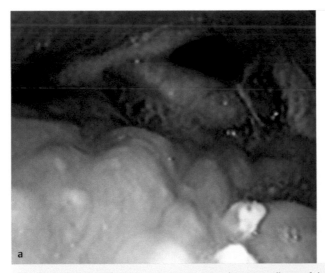 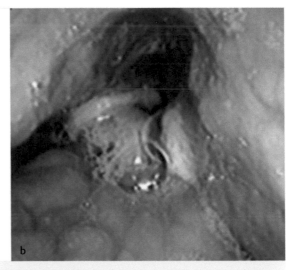

Fig. 16.1 **(a)** A partial anteroposterior EC, secondary to a collapse of the tongue base. **(b)** A complete anteroposterior EC, secondary to a collapse of the tongue base. Abbreviation: EC, epiglottic collapse.

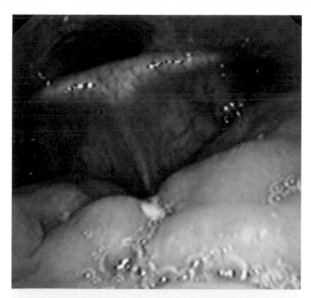

Fig. 16.2 An isolated anteroposterior EC. Abbreviation: EC, epiglottic collapse.

Besides conventional obstructive sleep apnea (OSA) treatment, several surgical techniques have been described in the literature to resolve an EC. Very few series have been published about indications, contraindications, techniques, success rates and complications of epiglottis surgery, and many sleep surgeons are reluctant to embark on epiglottis surgery anyhow, because of the risk of irreversible, permeant swallowing issues after partial epiglottectomy.[7,8,9] This particularly holds true for an isolated EC. It has to be said that the situation is essentially different in case of transoral robotic surgery (TORS) for severe OSA and CPAP failure, in which an EC is usually secondary to an AP collapse of the tongue base. Nevertheless, in TORS, a partial epiglottectomy, in addition to the robotic partial resection of tongue base, is performed as well. In such serious pathology, the risk of sequelae must be weighed differently in comparison with mild-to-moderate disease, where other treatment options might be more readily available. While it is known that after partial horizontal laryngectomy (in head and neck oncology), swallowing complications are often temporary, it is important to differentiate between sequelae of cancer surgery and benign disease. In mild-to-moderate OSA, other treatment options are available, and in severe OSA, invasive surgery is often offered as salvage therapy.

The finding of an EC is not rare, but its diagnosis requires invasive studies, since, as a rule, it cannot be established by indirect physical examination, flexible laryngoscopy, Müller maneuver, or imaging. The diagnosis of an EC has for long been felt as one of the important arguments in favor of performing DISE, since EC is a phenomenon that is exclusively detected during DISE. The recent development of performing DISE in different positions, as described in Chapter 11, has shed light on ECs, particularly isolated ECs. As described in Chapter 11, in our center, DISE is performed in different body positions, that is, in supine and lateral head (and trunk) rotation, and with and without applying jaw thrust. Based on observations made during DISE, we hypothesized that an isolated EC is, in particular, present in supine position and to a lesser extent when the patient is lying in a lateral body position. We were interested to see whether we could confirm our hypothesis by retrospectively analyzing if an isolated EC is more common in position-dependent OSA patients (PP) compared to nonpositional OSA patients (NPP) during DISE. Furthermore, we were interested in evaluating the impact of maneuvers and body position during DISE on an isolated EC, including jaw thrust, supine and lateral head (and trunk) position. The new insight is that an isolated EC almost exclusively occurs in supine position. In this chapter, we focus on the study performed to assess this phenomenon and its clinical implications.

16.2 Material and Methods

16.2.1 Patients

We performed a retrospective study, including a consecutive series of patients who underwent DISE at the Department of Otorhinolaryngology– Head and Neck Surgery of the OLVG (Amsterdam, The Netherlands) between August 2017 and August 2018. Among patients with sleep-disordered breathing (SDB), both nonapneic snoring patients and OSA patients were included. Patients were excluded when polysomnography (PSG) data concerning supine and nonsupine apnea–hypopnea index (AHI) and sleeping position was missing or when patients slept < 10% or > 90% of the total sleeping time (TST) in supine sleeping position, because subsequently supine or nonsupine AHI could not be determined reliably. Patients were also excluded when DISE results were inconclusive (e.g., due to mucosal hypersecretion) and could therefore not be interpreted.

16.2.2 Definitions

Patients were diagnosed with PP using Cartwright's criteria: a supine AHI of at least twice as high as nonsupine AHI.[10] As mentioned before, we were only interested in patients with a complete isolated AP EC, not secondary to a collapse of the tongue base, further referred to as a FE.

16.2.3 DISE Procedure

DISE was performed in a quiet outpatient endoscopy setting using propofol. The main reason to perform DISE was to evaluate surgical treatment options. Other indications included patients' eligibility for MAD treatment or combination therapy (e.g., MAD + positional therapy [PT]). DISE was performed by one experienced ENT resident (PV), with a trained nurse anesthetist managing sedation and monitoring blood pressure, electrocardiogram and oxygen levels. The level of sedation was controlled by a target-controlled infusion pump using the methods described by Schnider et al to calculate the effective dose.[11,12] Prior to the intravenous (IV) infusion of propofol, 2 mL Lidocaine was given IV to prevent pain caused by the infusion of propofol. In some patients, glycopyrrolate (Robinul) was given IV to prevent mucosal hypersecretion, since this could interfere with the quality of the endoscopic assessment.

16.2.4 Patient Positioning

Initially, DISE evaluation was commenced in supine position. Subsequently, the head was rotated to the lateral position, in order to mimic the effect of non-supine sleeping position.[20] Jaw thrust was performed in both positions to evaluate the effect of this maneuver on UA patency.

As described in Chapter 11 and in contrast to what was previously thought, the effect of lateral head rotation on UA patency in PP is not similar compared to both lateral head and trunk position.[13] As a result, in the period the study was running, we decided to modify the protocol. The DISE procedure remained unchanged in NPP, but in PP DISE, we adjusted the procedure by starting in lateral head and trunk position. After adequate evaluation, patients were maneuvered to supine head and trunk position. The jaw thrust was performed in both positions. The head was not rotated to the lateral position. Subsequently, results in NPP are presented using observations made in supine position and with the head rotated to

lateral position. In PP, results are described either using lateral head rotation or lateral head and trunk position.

16.3 Results

In total, 324 patients were included in this study. As many as 291 patients were diagnosed with OSA of which 72.5% (N = 211) were PP. The mean age was 48.4 ± 24.4 years, with a mean body mass index (BMI) of 27.1 ± 3.3 kg/m^2, median AHI of 17.7/h (8.3, 31.1), median supine AHI of 33.5/h (15.3, 56.6), and median nonsupine AHI of 7.1/h (2.8, 19.9). Patients spent a median percentage of the TST in supine position of 38.3% (25.9, 52.2), and the median oxygen desaturation index (ODI) was 19.8/h (10.3, 34.2). In PP, 19.4% were diagnosed with a FE compared to 16.8% in NPP, but no significant correlation was found between the presence of a FE and the presence of position dependency (p = 0.183). An overview of patient characteristics is given in ▶ Table 16.1.

16.3.1 DISE Findings

FE was found in supine position in 60 out of 324 patients (18.5%). Although we only focused on a FE, EC not secondary to an AC collapse of the tongue base, it was part of a multilevel problem (e.g., combined with a collapse at the level of the velum) in the majority of included patients. After applying a manual jaw thrust, aiming at 60 to 75% protrusion of the mandible, a FE was still present in 10 patients. When performing lateral head rotation in NPP, FE was no longer present in any of the patients. In PP, FE was still present in four patients when applying lateral head rotation only. In PP tilted to both lateral head and trunk rotation, a FE was found in only one subject. An overview of DISE findings can be found in ▶ Table 16.2.

Table 16.1 Baseline characteristics total population

Patient characteristic	Total N = 324	No OSA N = 33	NPP N = 80	PP N = 211	p value
Age (years)	48.4 ± 24.4	40.2 ± 10.0	48.3 ± 12.3	49.6 ± 28.8	0.688
Male/female	269/55	22/11	61/19	186/25	0.002*
BMI (kg/m^2)	27.1 ± 3.3	25.8 ± 3.6	27.2 ± 3.5	27.2 ± 3.5	0.991
Total AHI (events/h)	17.7 (8.3, 31.1)°	5.0 (2.0, 8.3)°	30.3 (15.9, 59.9)°	37.5 (22.6, 58.5)°	0.124
Non-supine AHI (events/h)	7.1 (2.8, 19.8)°	1.1 (0.6, 2.2)°	25.4 (10.4, 41.0)°	6.1 (2.8, 14.0)°	0.000*
TST in supine position (%)	40.2 ± 18.8	42.3 ± 18.0	42.6 ± 18.2	38.9 ± 19.1	0.134
ODI (events/h)	19.8 (10.3, 34.2)°	3.9 (2.7, 7.0)°	30.2 (15.1, 51.6)°	20.2 (12.3, 32.0)°	0.000*

Abbreviations: OSA, obstructive sleep apnea; NPP, non-positional obstructive sleep apnea patients; PP, positional obstructive sleep apnea patients; BMI, body mass index; AHI, apnea–hypopnea index; TST, total sleeping time; ODI, oxygen desaturation index.
Note: Data presented as mean ± standard deviation or °median (Q1, Q3). *p value < 0.05 comparing NPP and PP.

Table 16.2 Overview of the presence of a FE in different body positions, with and without maneuvers in patients with no OSA, NPP and PP

Patient characteristic	FE	No FE	FE vs no FE p value
Number (%)	60 (18.5)	264 (81.5)	48 vs 228
Age (years)	47.5 ± 11.9	48.6 ± 26.4	0.756
Male/female	53/7	216/48	0.914
BMI (kg/m^2)	27.0 ± 3.6	27.1 ± 3.3	0.787
Total AHI (events/h)	14.4 (8.2, 25.0)°	18.3 (8.3, 32.4)°	0.317
Supine AHI (events/h)	28.9 (14.3, 56.6)°	35.0 (15.5, 57.0)°	0.260
Non-supine AHI (events/h)	5.9 (2.7, 16.0)°	8.1 (2.8, 20.1)°	0.173
TST in supine position (%)	41.1 (28.2, 63.1)°	37.6 (25.8, 51.5)°	0.475
ODI (events/h)	20.0 (10.2, 31.3)°	19.8 (10.3, 34.8)°	0.949

Abbreviations: BMI, body mass index; AHI, apnea–hypopnea index; TST, total sleeping time; ODI, oxygen desaturation index; FE, floppy epiglottis; NPP, nonpositional OSA; OSA, obstruction sleep apnea; PP, positional OSA.
Note: Data presented as mean ± standard deviation or °median (Q1, Q3). *p value < 0.05

16.4 Discussion

The results of this study indicate that a FE appears almost exclusively in supine body position and to a lesser extent during lateral head (and trunk) rotation. Despite this observation, the prevalence of a FE was similar in NPP and PP. Neither could we find a significant correlation between the presence of FE and position-dependency.

This could be explained by the fact that in this study, we did not exclude patients with a FE as part of a multilevel collapse observed during DISE.

In total, only two patients were identified with isolated FE, meaning that no collapse was found at the level of the velum, oropharynx and tongue base.

Interestingly enough, those two patients were phenotypically different: they were younger, had a low BMI, and had a supine AHI twice as high as the nonsupine AHI. These characteristics are comparable to those of PP.[14,15,16,17]

The findings of this study are supported by several previously published articles. First, Marques et al observed 23 OSA patients who underwent an UA endoscopy during natural sleep to evaluate the effect of sleeping position and the correlation with pharyngeal structures involved in UA collapse. Additional recordings of airflow and pharyngeal pressure were simultaneously executed. EC was found in six patients who showed substantial improvement in UA patency when turned to lateral body position. Objective measurements also showed a decrease in percentage of breaths exhibiting EC (from 66.5 to 12.3%) and an increase in ventilation by 45%, comparing supine to lateral body position.[18]

In addition, another study showed a positive effect of changing body position on UA patency in EC.[19] These results were confirmed by a third study, in which lateral head rotation was associated with a decrease in EC compared to supine position.[20]

As previously mentioned in this chapter, diagnosis of an EC requires invasive studies such as DISE. In literature, less invasive diagnostic tools to identify airflow patterns and its relation to the underlying structures involved in UA collapse have been proposed. One of these alternatives has been previously described by Azarbarzin et al. They analyzed flow characteristics correlated with the presence of FE and concluded that this type of UA collapse was associated with flow features, characterized by discontinuity and jaggedness.[21] Unfortunately, these algorithms are not externally validated or yet part of daily practice.

16.5 Conclusion

The results of this study indicate that a FE is a position-dependent phenomenon, which appears almost exclusively in supine body position. Despite this phenomenon, the correlation with the underlying pathophysiological mechanism in NPP and PP remains unclear to date.

16.6 Clinical Relevance

Treatment of OSA patients with a FE remains challenging, since both conservative and surgical treatment is hampered by low conservative treatment success rate and possible complications accompanied with surgical interventions.

It can be concluded that there is a demand for other treatment options in patients with this type of UA collapse. Based on the results of this study, avoiding the supine sleep position is a rational advice. Recent developments have shown that PT with new-generation devices are effective in reducing the percentage of supine sleep in PP.[22,23,24,25] In addition, PT in patients a FE might be a promising alternative as a standalone treatment or in combination with other treatment modalities, for example, less invasive forms of UA surgery of the other levels of UA obstruction, limiting risks and complications.

References

[1] Kezirian EJ, Hohenhorst W, de Vries N. Drug-induced sleep endoscopy: the VOTE classification. Eur Arch Otorhinolaryngol. 2011; 268 (8):1233–1236

[2] Torre C, Camacho M, Liu SY, Huon LK, Capasso R. Epiglottis collapse in adult obstructive sleep apnea: a systematic review. Laryngoscope. 2016; 126(2):515–523

[3] Verse T, Pirsig W. Age-related changes in the epiglottis causing failure of nasal continuous positive airway pressure therapy. J Laryngol Otol. 1999; 113(11):1022–1025

[4] Dedhia RC, Rosen CA, Soose RJ. What is the role of the larynx in adult obstructive sleep apnea? Laryngoscope. 2014; 124(4):1029–1034

[5] Shimohata T, Tomita M, Nakayama H, Aizawa N, Ozawa T, Nishizawa M. Floppy epiglottis as a contraindication of CPAP in patients with multiple system atrophy. Neurology. 2011; 76(21):1841–1842

[6] Kent DT, Rogers R, Soose RJ. Drug-induced sedation endoscopy in the evaluation of OSA patients with incomplete oral appliance therapy response. Otolaryngol Head Neck Surg. 2015; 153(2):302–307

[7] Catalfumo FJ, Golz A, Westerman ST, Gilbert LM, Joachims HZ, Goldenberg D. The epiglottis and obstructive sleep apnoea syndrome. J Laryngol Otol. 1998; 112(10):940–943

[8] Golz A, Goldenberg D, Westerman ST, et al. Laser partial epiglottidectomy as a treatment for obstructive sleep apnea and laryngomalacia. Ann Otol Rhinol Laryngol. 2000; 109(12 Pt 1):1140–1145

[9] Bourolias C, Hajiioannou J, Sobol E, Velegrakis G, Helidonis E. Epiglottis reshaping using CO2 laser: a minimally invasive technique and its potent applications. Head Face Med. 2008; 4:15

[10] Cartwright RD. Effect of sleep position on sleep apnea severity. Sleep. 1984; 7(2):110–114

[11] Schnider T, Minto C. Pharmacokinetic models of propofol for TCI. Anaesthesia. 2008; 63(2):206–206, author reply 206–207

[12] Schnider TW, Minto CF, Gambus PL, et al. The influence of method of administration and covariates on the pharmacokinetics of propofol in adult volunteers. Anesthesiology. 1998; 88(5):1170–1182

[13] Vonk PE, van de Beek MJ, Ravesloot MJL, de Vries N. Drug-induced sleep endoscopy: new insights in lateral head rotation compared to lateral head and trunk rotation in (non)positional obstructive sleep apnea patients. Laryngoscope. 2019; 129(10):2430–2435

[14] Ravesloot MJ, Frank MH, van Maanen JP, Verhagen EA, de Lange J, de Vries N. Positional OSA part 2: retrospective cohort analysis with a new classification system (APOC). Sleep Breath. 2016; 20(2):881–888

[15] Richard W, Kox D, den Herder C, Laman M, van Tinteren H, de Vries N. The role of sleep position in obstructive sleep apnea syndrome. Eur Arch Otorhinolaryngol. 2006; 263(10):946–950

[16] Oksenberg A, Silverberg DS, Arons E, Radwan H. Positional vs nonpositional obstructive sleep apnea patients: anthropomorphic, nocturnal polysomnographic, and multiple sleep latency test data. Chest. 1997; 112(3):629–639

[17] Itasaka Y, Miyazaki S, Ishikawa K, Togawa K. The influence of sleep position and obesity on sleep apnea. Psychiatry Clin Neurosci. 2000; 54(3):340–341

[18] Marques M, Genta PR, Sands SA, et al. Effect of sleeping position on upper airway patency in obstructive sleep apnea is determined by the pharyngeal structure causing collapse. Sleep (Basel). 2017; 40(3)

[19] Victores AJ, Hamblin J, Gilbert J, Switzer C, Takashima M. Usefulness of sleep endoscopy in predicting positional obstructive sleep apnea. Otolaryngol Head Neck Surg. 2014; 150(3):487–493

[20] Safiruddin F, Koutsourelakis I, de Vries N. Analysis of the influence of head rotation during drug-induced sleep endoscopy in obstructive sleep apnea. Laryngoscope. 2014; 124(9):2195–2199

[21] Azarbarzin A, Marques M, Sands SA, et al. Predicting epiglottic collapse in patients with obstructive sleep apnoea. Eur Respir J. 2017; 50(3):1700345

[22] Benoist LB, Verhagen M, Torensma B, van Maanen JP, de Vries N. Positional therapy in patients with residual positional obstructive sleep apnea after upper airway surgery. Sleep Breath. 2016; 21(2): 279–288

[23] van Maanen JP, de Vries N. Long-term effectiveness and compliance of positional therapy with the sleep position trainer in the treatment of positional obstructive sleep apnea syndrome. Sleep (Basel). 2014; 37(7):1209–1215

[24] van Maanen JP, Meester KA, Dun LN, et al. The sleep position trainer: a new treatment for positional obstructive sleep apnoea. Sleep Breath. 2013; 17(2):771–779

[25] Ravesloot MJL, White D, Heinzer R, Oksenberg A, Pépin JL. Efficacy of the new generation of devices for positional therapy for patients with positional obstructive sleep apnea: a systematic review of the literature and meta-analysis. J Clin Sleep Med. 2017; 13(6):813–824

17 Common Mistakes in DISE

Filippo Montevecchi, Giovanni Cammaroto, and Riccardo Gobbi

Abstract

In this chapter, the authors describe all the possible mistakes during drug-induced sleep endoscopy (DISE), reviewing the international literature and discussing more than 10 years of experience in this field of sleep medicine.

Keywords: mistakes, DISE, sleep endoscopy, sleep medicine

17.1 Introduction

Drug-induced sleep endoscopy (DISE) is a fiberoptic examination of the upper airways (UA) under controlled sedation, performed to determine the exact site(s) of UA' collapse in patients with sleep-disordered breathing (SDB).

Quantifying the location and identifying the mechanisms of UA collapse with DISE may potentially help to tailor surgical treatments and improve their outcomes.

Many physicians believe that performing DISE can solve all dilemmas in patients affected by obstructive sleep apnea (OSA) but this is certainly a common mistake. This examination can provide several significant pieces of information but there are different possible variables that may lead to misunderstandings.

In 1991, Croft and Pringle[1] described an original way to study OSA patients, the "sleep nasoendoscopy," a procedure designed to observe the UA under pharmacologically induced sleep. At that time, the main criticism seemed to be related to a substantial difference between natural physiological sleep and induced sleep during DISE. Numerous studies have subsequently looked at sleep architecture during sedation to demonstrate differences and similarities.[2] The depth of sedation was questioned, as different degrees of obstruction would be observed, depending on the depth of sedation. A more objective measurement of sleep depth is now possible by means of bispectral index monitoring (BIS, Medtronic. Minneapolis, MN, USA), recently introduced in advanced DISE settings instead of simple clinical judgment (patient's capability to react to different verbal and tactile stimuli).

Few studies demonstrate that overall observer agreement was higher in experienced versus nonexperienced ENT surgeons, suggesting that experience in performing DISE is necessary to obtain reliable observations. Training under guidance of an experienced surgeon, and the use of advanced setting technologies (target-controlled infusion (TCI), sleep depth measurement and online cardiorespiratory monitoring), might be helpful for unexperienced physicians.[3] In the last two decades, DISE has become of increasing interest in the medical community, as evidenced by the significant number of articles concerning its use and its worldwide spread.

17.2 Setting and Preoperative Investigations

Performing a sleep study (at least a type III polysomnography [PSG]) before DISE is considered mandatory. If a sleep study is not available, the physician is not able to score the degree of OSA and understand certain features, such as positionality, that should be known before performing DISE.

In our institution, patients undergo propofol-induced DISE in the operating room, with standard monitoring and availability of resuscitation equipment. The constant use of a specific drug helps in the understanding of its effects in OSA patients and standardizes the procedure. Therefore, the use of different drugs may lead to heterogeneous data. Patients are positioned supine in a bed with or without pillow according to the habits of the patient. A possible mistake is performing DISE without all the anesthesiology equipment: OSA patients' airways may be difficult to manage, especially when severe oxygen desaturations and degrees of collapse are needed to better understand the mechanisms of OSA. DISE should reproduce as much as possible the sleep features registered during PSG, in particular oxygen desaturation during non REM sleep, in order to obtain reliable findings.

Another error involves performing DISE on a surgical bed. The use of a conventional bed may help to better reproduce physiological sleep.

Topical anesthetics are not used for the nasal or pharyngeal mucosa, nor are any drying agents. Any kind of topical drugs used can change the physiological behavior of the UA.

A nasal fiberscope is used for visualization and measurements at three anatomic levels: the velopharynx or retropalatal (RP) region, hypopharynx or retroglossal (RG) region, and retroepiglottic (RE) region. A bulky endoscope may awake or disturb the patient during the examination, therefore pediatric instruments are preferred.

Finally, a quiet and dark room appears to be the best environment for an effective examination.

17.3 Technical Equipment

In order to perform DISE correctly, it would be preferable to use specific technical equipment. Standard monitoring (SaO_2, ECG, Blood Pressure), TCI for anesthetic drugs (not available in USA), Bispectral (BIS) index, video and audio recording and simultaneous cardiorespiratory monitoring for selected cases (represent the most updated suggested setting). It is not possible to perform a DISE without, at least, standard monitoring.

In OSA patients, the observation of apneic events is imperative for diagnostic accuracy, especially for patients possibly undergoing a tailored surgical therapy.

DISE performed with TCI technique should be the first choice because of its increased accuracy, stability and safety in comparison with the bolus technique. Manual infusion may cause an inadequate and unsettled brain concentration of the sedative agent if the anesthesiologist administers it too quickly.[4]

17.4 Patient Positioning and Diagnostic Maneuvers

It has already been mentioned that during DISE patients are positioned supine on a bed with or without pillow according to the habits of the patient. Transnasal fiberoptic endoscopy has to be performed in awake patients and during sedation. It is suggested to know the anatomy of the UA before sedation to facilitate the introduction of the fiberscope and avoid discomfort and awakening of the patient.

A transoral endoscopy is also recommended to better evaluate a velar collapse and distinguish a primary from a secondary collapse. Transoral endoscopy allows to highlight if the oral tongue pushes the soft palate back, and therefore understand if the collapse is secondary. This maneuver should be better performed using a protection (e.g., Guedel airway insertion or a metallic ear speculum) to protect the instrument.

The jaw lift maneuver during transnasal endoscopy allows to evaluate if the space behind the soft palate may increase. By performing this maneuver, it is possible to understand if an oral appliance, or an alternative a maxillo-mandibular advancement, can be suggested to treat an OSA patient. The main mistake during this maneuver is to pull the mandible too anteriorly. It is important to implement in DISE routine the use of a mandibular advancement device (MAD) simulator instead of jaw lift because of its more reliable outcomes.[5]

Another common mistake is not evaluating the UA with opened and closed mouth. This maneuver allows the physician to understand if the patient can benefit from nasal treatments or an oral appliance.

Rotating the head and/or positioning patients on one side may also provide information on OSA positionality and lead to other therapeutic options.

17.5 Observation Window

One of the most frequent errors during DISE is to check the UA too early or too late during the sedation.

In the beginning of the procedure, it is common to notice both unstable breathing and central apneas, with complete UA obstruction. Clinical experience in DISE or the use of advanced monitoring (PSG type III) should help in avoiding common mistakes.

It is important to observe at least two or more cycles of snoring and/or collapses for each segment of the UA (cycle definition: a complete and stable sequence of snoring–obstructing hypo/apnea– oxygen desaturation– breathing). The lowest oxygen saturation (LOS) reached during the procedure should be close to the LOS registered in the sleep study. If BIS is available in our setting, a score of around 50 to 70 allows to reach an appropriate degree of sedation.

Beginning DISE by observing the tongue base first is another frequent mistake. It is advisable to study the velum and then the tongue base, because the scope can modify the collapse, working like a stent at the velum level.[6]

17.6 Target Events

The following events should be observed during DISE:
- Snoring, interpreted as pharyngeal and/or laryngeal vibration.
- Apnea, intended as partial (>75%) or complete obstruction.
- Type of collapse pattern (lateral, anteroposterior [AP], or circumferential).

Hypopneas may be difficult to evaluate, as they consist of partial obstruction of UA; online cardiorespiratory monitoring not only helps in detecting these events but also aids in defining the specific kind of apnea (obstructive, mixed, or central).[7]

A retrospective study on 250 consecutive patients, making a comparison between awake and DISE findings, was published in 2010.[8] In this study, significant differences between hypopharyngeal degree and pattern of obstruction (59% and 49%, respectively) were found and up to 30% of cases, observed by DISE, presented with laryngeal obstruction; epiglottic obstruction was classified as primary if the collapse was produced by intrinsic instability of the larynx and secondary if the tongue base or the lateral wall were responsible for the supraglottic collapse. Endoscopic findings are essential to guide the surgical decision-making. It has to be acknowledged that awake endoscopy may frequently underestimate the degree of the hypopharyngeal and laryngeal obstruction.

Finally, few neurological diseases may mimic some benign SDB. For instance, laryngeal stridor can be easily confused with simple snoring. Stridor is a harsh, high-pitched, musical sound produced by turbulent airflow through a partially obstructed airway. Nocturnal stridor is produced by obstruction on the glottis level and is often associated to multiple system atrophy, a disease with decreased survival.

17.7 Classification System

The use of a classification system for DISE appears to be fundamental. Whatever diagnostic tool we decide to use, one of the main problems encountered is the standardization of the description of the sites and dynamic patterns of UA collapses. There is no consensus regarding which scoring system should be utilized to report findings during DISE. The VOTE system[9] and NOHL classification[10] are the most frequent scoring systems reported for patients undergoing DISE. The latest update of the European position paper in DISE decided to adopt velum, oropharynx, tongue base, and epiglottis (VOTE) classification as essential with the possibility of adding comments (e.g., anatomical structures involved in the obstruction) for each level in order to have a common starting dataset and results.[11]

Classification system in OSA patients, representing a simple, quick, and effective diagnostic tool and its application, especially for decision-making and analysis of surgical outcomes, is strongly recommended. Standardization of the reporting of DISE findings would also improve comparability among studies.

17.8 Counseling after DISE

Discussing DISE findings with patients is surely one of the most critical phases.

Pros and cons of the proposed therapeutic alternatives need to be clarified, especially focusing on the possible success rate of each treatment. Ventilation therapy should be always taken into consideration, being the most successful treatment described in literature.

17.9 Conclusion

Today, alternative treatments to ventilation have become increasingly required. In order to obtain satisfactory surgical outcomes, an accurate UA evaluation and careful patient selection are mandatory. Scientific community is still looking for the ideal technique for evaluating UA obstruction. DISE, however, remains one of the best tools for studying OSA patients before opting for alternative treatments such as surgical interventions. Anyway, it is important to remember that technical and clinical mistakes can be made in all stages of this advanced diagnostic procedure.

References

[1] Croft CB, Pringle M. Sleep nasendoscopy: a technique of assessment in snoring and obstructive sleep apnoea. Clin Otolaryngol Allied Sci. 1991; 16(5):504–509

[2] Rabelo FA, Küpper DS, Sander HH, Fernandes RM, Valera FC. Polysomnographic evaluation of propofol-induced sleep in patients with respiratory sleep disorders and controls. Laryngoscope. 2013; 123 (9):2300–2305

[3] Vroegop AV, Vanderveken OM, Wouters K, et al. Observer variation in drug-induced sleep endoscopy: experienced versus nonexperienced ear, nose, and throat surgeons. Sleep (Basel). 2013; 36(6):947–953

[4] De Vito A, Agnoletti V, Berrettini S, et al. Drug-induced sleep endoscopy: conventional versus target controlled infusion techniques—a randomized controlled study. Eur Arch Otorhinolaryngol. 2011; 268 (3):457–462

[5] Vroegop AV, Vanderveken OM, Dieltjens M, et al. Sleep endoscopy with simulation bite for prediction of oral appliance treatment outcome. J Sleep Res. 2013; 22(3):348–355

[6] De Vito A, Carrasco Llatas M, Vanni A, et al. European position paper on drug-induced sedation endoscopy (DISE). Sleep Breath. 2014; 18 (3):453–465

[7] Gobbi R, Baiardi S, Mondini S, et al. Technique and preliminary analysis of drug-induced sleep endoscopy with online polygraphic cardiorespiratory monitoring in patients with obstructive sleep apnea syndrome. JAMA Otolaryngol Head Neck Surg. 2017; 143(5):459–465

[8] Campanini A, Canzi P, De Vito A, Dallan I, Montevecchi F, Vicini C. Awake versus sleep endoscopy: personal experience in 250 OSAHS patients. Acta Otorhinolaryngol Ital. 2010; 30(2):73–77

[9] Kezirian EJ, Hohenhorst W, de Vries N. Drug-induced sleep endoscopy: the VOTE classification. Eur Arch Otorhinolaryngol. 2011; 268 (8):1233–1236

[10] Vicini C, De Vito A, Benazzo M, et al. The nose oropharynx hypopharynx and larynx (NOHL) classification: a new system of diagnostic standardized examination for OSAHS patients. Eur Arch Otorhinolaryngol. 2012; 269(4):1297–1300

[11] De Vito A, Carrasco Llatas M, Ravesloot MJ, et al. European position paper on drug-induced sleep endoscopy: 2017 Update. Clin Otolaryngol. 2018; 43(6):1541–1552

18 Diagnostic and Therapeutic Applications or a Guide for Clinical Practice

Clemens Heiser and Joachim T. Maurer

Abstract

Drug-induced sleep endoscopy (DISE) and hypoglossal nerve stimulation (HNS).

HNS has become increasingly important in the treatment of patients with obstructive sleep apnea (OSA) over the last few years. It is the first therapy, especially in breathing-synchronized selective HNS, where DISE has been shown to increase the clinical results after implantation. Nowadays, DISE plays a crucial part in the selection of the patients for HNS. Therefore, this chapter summarizes the most important topics, which need to be known for screening patients with DISE for HNS.

Keywords: hypoglossal nerve stimulation, upper airway stimulation, obstructive sleep apnea, palatoglossal coupling, drug-induced sleep endoscopy, surgical alternatives

18.1 History

18.1.1 History about Hypoglossal Nerve Stimulation

During the last few years, HNS—also known as upper airway stimulation (UAS)—has been proven to be effective in patients with obstructive sleep apnea (OSA), who are not compliant or adherent to continuous positive airway pressure (CPAP).[1,2,3,4,5] Even on a long-term follow-up after 3 and 5 years of implantation, improvements in sleepiness, quality of life, and respiratory outcomes are observed.[6,7] Almost no serious events related to the implantation of the system or its regular use have been reported, which allows the conclusion that this surgical treatment has long-term benefits for individuals with moderate-to-severe OSA.[7] Different systems have been developed during the last two decades.[8] The main target of these stimulation systems is the HN. Different technical approaches, which are wholly available in the markets in Europe and partly available in the USA, help to achieve this aim:

- Breathing-synchronized selective stimulation (Inspire Medical Systems Maple Grove, MN, USA), which has a CE labeling and FDA approval.[9]
- Nonbreathing-synchronized continuous stimulation (ImThera Medical, San Diego, CA, USA), which has a CE labeling but no FDA approval.[10]

Other stimulation systems are currently under development, such as a bilateral stimulation system for selective stimulation of the HN, which receives energy pulses from an external power source (Nyxoah Genio System, Mont-St-Guibert, Belgium).[11]

All of these therapeutic stimulation applications have been developed by using neuromuscular electrical stimulation of the HN, mainly activating the genioglossus muscle. These techniques are powerful alternatives to CPAP or other upper airway (UA) surgical procedures. The HNS therapies consist of an implanted, programmable neurostimulation system, with a stimulation electrode around the HN. The breathingcycle-synchronized system selectively stimulates the distal medial branches of the HN, which are mainly responsible for protruding the tongue.[12,13,14,15,16] The stimulation period is adjusted by the physician using a programmer and delivering the stimulation during the late expiratory phase and throughout the entire inspiratory phase of respiration.[17,18] Furthermore, different stimulation settings, such as amplitude, pulse rate and width, and electrode configuration are set by the physician during nighttime titration in the sleep laboratory. DISE plays a crucial role in the patient selection for this therapy. The nonbreathing-synchronized stimulation places the stimulation electrode around the main trunk of the HN.[19,20] The cuff electrode consists of six circular contacts, which depolarize sectors of the main nerve trunk, which can be sequentially activated and programmed independently. This allows continuous stimulation during both inspiration and expiration, and a respiration sensor electrode is not required. For this system, patient selection seems to be easier than the breathing-synchronized system because no DISE is required during the screening process.[10]

18.1.2 History about DISE in Selective HN Stimulation—The Key Factor to Success

As already described above, DISE plays an important role during the patient selection in breathing-synchronized selective stimulation compared to nonbreathing-synchronized continuous stimulation.[21,22] When the first clinical trials started in selective HNS, the main basic clinical trial revealed that patients with a complete concentric collapse at the soft palate have a high risk of being nonresponders to therapy.[21] A total of 21 patients with OSA, who underwent an implantation of a breathing-synchronized stimulation system (Inspire Medical Systems Maple Grove, MN, USA), received a DISE before surgery. Afterward, 16 patients were identified without complete concentric collapse at the soft palate, and their apnea–hypopnea index (AHI) reduced from 37.6 ± 11.4/h to 11.6 ± 11.7/h. Five patients who showed complete concentric collapse at the soft palate before surgery during DISE did not have a significant change in AHI with UAS 6 months after implantation, as baseline AHI was 41.5 ± 13.8/h and AHI with UAS was 48.1 ± 18.7/h.[21] The authors concluded that the absence of a palatal complete concentric collapse during DISE may predict therapeutic success with implanted UAS therapy. During the following Phase III and IV trials in international prospective multicenter settings, using this in addition to other inclusion criteria, the success rate could be much improved.[1,3,4] The STAR trial revealed a median AHI score from 29.3/h to 9.0/h at 12 months.[1] The German postmarket study in a commercial setting strengthened the evidence that the treatment can be successfully transferred from the controlled trial setting into routine clinical practice.[3] The median AHI was again significantly reduced at 6 months from 28.6/h to 8.3/h[3]. DISE was the crucial part of patient selection in all of these clinical trials. Previous trials not using DISE criteria revealed that HNS in nonselected OSA patients leads to increased interindividual variation and reduced predictability regarding therapeutic effectiveness.[23,24,25,26,27]

18.2 Hypoglossal Nerve Anatomy

Both the human tongue and HN play crucial roles in the anatomical pathophysiology of OSA.[28,29] The tongue muscle groups can be divided into retractors (styloglossus and hyoglossus muscles) and protrusors (genioglossus muscle) with its intrinsic tongue stiffeners (transverse and vertical muscles).[15,29] Furthermore, the geniohyoid muscle, which does not actually belong to the tongue muscles, and is innervated by the first cervical spinal nerve, moves the hyoid forward and helps to open the UA at the hypopharyngeal level.[15] The genioglossus horizontal, which is the most inferior portion of the genioglossus muscle, also inserts on the hyoid bone and contributes to moving the hyoid forward. ▸ Fig. 18.1 gives an overview of the HN and the different tongue muscles. Different phenotypes have been described and a classification system of the nerves has been developed.[15]

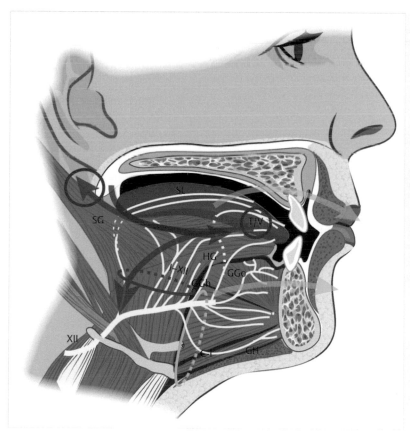

Fig. 18.1 Schematic drawing of the different muscle groups and their innervations by the different fibers of the hypoglossal nerve (XII). The green circle indicates the fibers, which are protruding the tongue and need to be included in the stimulation lead. The red circle indicates the lateral fibers of the hypoglossal nerve, which need to be excluded. Stimulation of T/V leads to an activation of the palatoglossus muscle, which helps to open the soft palate (purple arrow, palatoglossus coupling).
Abbreviations: SG, styloglossus muscle; HG, hyoglossus muscle; SL, superior longitudinal; GH, geniohyoid muscle; T/V, intrinsic vertical and horizontal muscle fibers; GGo, genioglossus muscle oblique; GGh, genioglossus muscle horizontal; l–XII, lateral fibers of the hypoglossal nerve (XII), m–XII, medial fibers of the hypoglossal nerve (XII); XII, hypoglossal nerve.

18.3 Pathophysiology and Mechanisms of Stimulation

18.3.1 Anatomical Pattern and Level of Obstructions in the Pathophysiology of OSA

Targeting surgical treatment of OSA requires identification of the level and pattern of obstructions during sleep.[30,31] Unfortunately, endoscopy of the UA during natural sleep is neither feasible nor reliable due to sleep-disturbing effects of the endoscopic examination. Since Croft and Pringle first described DISE in 1991, patterns and levels of obstructions could be assessed.[32] The next important step was the investigations of Eastwood et al, who demonstrated a correlation between propensity for collapse of the UA during sleep and under general anesthesia.[33] Nowadays, the conduct of DISE has been much improved, due to UAS also. Protocols have been developed for reliable results.[34] Obstruction can occur at different levels of the pharynx[35]:

- Velum.
- Oropharynx.
- Tongue base.
- Epiglottis.

Other locations for obstructions are extremely rare and have been described with other classification systems such as nose, oropharynx, hypopharynx, and larynx (NOHL) compared to the most commonly used velum, oropharynx, tongue base, and epiglottis (VOTE).[30,35,36] However, the level of obstruction is not the only important consideration when selecting the appropriate surgical procedure, as the pattern and degree of obstruction are also significant.[22] In further studies, complete concentric collapse could be shown to be compatible, because the patient population was so small in feasibility studies (▶ Fig. 18.2a, **Video 9**). ▶ Table 18.1 provides an overview of obstructions which can be detected during DISE, probably affecting the outcome of UAS. It is known that UAS is not only affecting the tongue base by stimulating the main tongue nerve but also protruding the tongue.[18,22] The whole UA is affected by this stimulation due to interconnecting muscle fibers, which helps to open the level of the velum too.[37] In the following section, the probable mechanisms and its effects on the different anatomic levels during stimulation are discussed.

Velum

In the late 1990s, Ferguson et al could show that oral appliances can increase the diameter at the soft palate.[38] It seems to be that a maximal advancement of the mandible is needed to obtain therapeutic effects in patients with OSA; meanwhile, a lesser degree of tongue protrusion may also be effective. But the effect on the velopharyngeal level

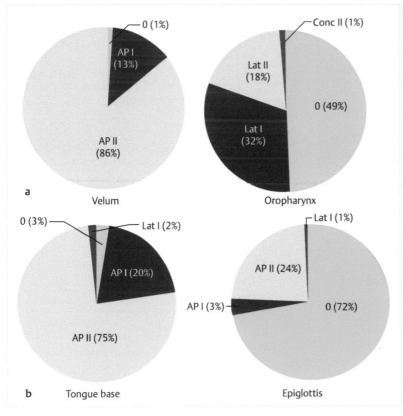

Fig. 18.2 (a, b) Showing the different obstruction patterns and levels in 100 OSA patients with breath-synchronized hypoglossal nerve stimulation before surgery. Abbreviations: 0, no obstruction; AP, anteroposterior; Lat, lateral; Conc, concentric.

Table 18.1 Overview obstruction levels and patterns regarding VOTE classification[35]

	Pattern	Maneuver	Recommendation	Maneuver	Recommendation
Velum	**AP**	**Yes**	**Strong**	No	Weak–strong
Velum	Lateral	Yes	Weak–strong	No	Caution
Velum	Concentric	Yes	Weak	*No*	*Contra*
Orolateral pharyngeal wall	Lateral with tonsils hyperplasia	Yes	Caution (tonsillectomy first and reevaluate)	No	Caution (tonsillectomy first and reevaluate)
Orolateral pharyngeal wall	Lateral without hyperplasia of the tonsils	Yes	Weak	No	Contra–caution
Tongue Base	**AP**	**Yes**	**Strong**	No	Weak
Epiglottis	**AP**	**Yes**	**Strong**	No	Weak
Epiglottis	Lateral	Yes	Strong	No	Weak

Abbreviation: HNS, hypoglossal nerve stimulation.

Note: Different collapse patterns can occur at the different anatomic levels. Different combinations of obstruction levels and patterns are shown in this table. Maneuver is chin lift or Esmarch maneuver, marked with "yes" or "no," if the obstruction levels open during this maneuver. The recommendations are given in a gradual manner, starting with the strongest to the lowest as follows: strong–weak–caution–contra. The most favorable obstruction levels and patterns are set in bold and the contraindications for selective HNS are set in italics.

seems to vary from one patient to another, even in HNS.[22] Today, it is known that selective UAS also has an effect on the obstruction pattern at the soft palate. This effect on the velum during stimulation can be explained by palatoglossal coupling.[37] The palatoglossal muscle runs from the soft palate to the tongue base in the anterior palatal pillar (▶ Fig. 18.1).[39,40] This muscle acts like an anchor, which passively opens the velum when the tongue is moved forward. Another explanation for this mechanism may be that as the tongue is moved forward, the pressure on the soft palate may be relieved and the velum can remain open.[37] A third theory includes the movement of the hyoid arch, where pharyngeal muscles and ligaments are connected.[41] A movement forward is associated with glossopharyngeal breathing, whereby air is first gulped into the oropharynx through the nose, and then pushed into lungs.[42,43] To understand the exact mechanism further, research projects are needed. It is also conceivable that an interaction between the different pathophysiological models occurs, and on the other hand, pathophysiology differs from patient to another. But what all three models have in common is that an unhindered stiffened elongated tongue is needed to relieve the burden on the soft palate. Therefore, the stimulation lead needs to include the transverse and vertical fibers of the HN, which are responsible for the intrinsic muscles.[15,37] This stabilizing effect on the soft palate also explains why patients with an AP collapse at this level benefit most from HNS.

Lateral Oropharyngeal Wall

The lateral walls of the pharynx, consisting mainly of the tonsils, are an important component of some patients' collapse patterns. A hyperplasia of the tonsils (Friedman size 3 or 4) should be the indication for a tonsillectomy combined with surgery of the soft palate (e.g., uvulopalatopharyngoplasty).[44,45] In cases of severe lateral pharyngeal wall collapse during DISE, one should be extremely cautious regarding the indication for HNS. Lateral collapse patterns can worsen by moving the tongue forward. A chin lift or Esmarch maneuver can be a very helpful tool during DISE, providing the surgeon with a partial impression of what might happen during stimulation.[46] An indirect effect of the constrictor muscles, which form the lateral walls in the pharynx, can be explained by the hyoid arch movement.[41] Moving the hyoid forward, where the middle pharyngeal constrictor is connected, can close the UA on the lateral oropharyngeal wall level. Further research projects are needed to understand the pathophysiological mechanisms and physiological *settings* at this level during stimulation.

Tongue Base

The main opener of the entire UA and tongue base is the genioglossus muscle as described above.[47,48,49] It is one of the paired extrinsic muscles of the tongue, which is mainly responsible for protruding the tongue forward.[28,29,50] The muscle comprises two compartments. The oblique compartment pulls the tongue body downward and the horizontal compartment pulls the tongue base and hyoid forward.[15,28] All stimulation systems, which are currently on the market or under development, are targeting this muscle.[17,51] This main airway opener plays a crucial role in the pathophysiology and treatment options. AP collapse during DISE and related possible explanatory approaches in these patients for their sleep apnea are good candidates for HNS.

Epiglottis

The epiglottis is connected to the hyoid bone. Simultaneously, the hyoid bone provides attachment to the muscles of the floor of the mouth (mylohyoid muscle), muscles of the tongue above (hyoglossus muscle), muscles to the larynx below, and muscles to the pharynx posterior (middle pharyngeal constrictor). Furthermore, it is important to know that the geniohyoid muscle, which is a narrow muscle, runs from the chin to the superior, medial border of the hyoid bone.[15,29] It brings the hyoid bone forward and upward. This helps to dilate the UA during breathing.[52] This muscle is innervated by fibers from the first cervical nerve (C1) which travels alongside the HN.[18] When including C1 in the stimulation lead during selective breathing-synchronized HNS, the contraction of the geniohyoid muscle leads to an "active" anterior hyoid displacement and in addition moves the epiglottis forward. Therefore, it is highly recommended to identify C1 during surgery and include it in the stimulation lead.[15,18,53,54,55] Thus, obstructions on the epiglottic level may be resolved by HNS and are not an exclusion criterion for this unique alternative treatment.

18.4 DISE in HNS as a Screening Tool—Procedure for Best Practice

To obtain a reliable result in the screening process for selective breathing-synchronized HNS, it is critical to standardize the DISE procedure. We developed a protocol which should be part of the selection in OSA patients and is described as follows[34,56]:

DISE can be performed in the setting of an operating or recovery room, which is dark, silent, and climate-controlled to reduce adverse external stimuli during the procedure. Standard anesthesia monitoring including resuscitation equipment and a monitored recovery facility should be nearby. Vital parameters are recorded. The level of sedation should be controlled by measuring entropy or bispectral index score (BIS).[57,58] During the entire procedure, vital parameters are measured as follows: three-channel electrocardiogram (ECG), pulse oximetry, and noninvasive blood pressure every 10 minutes.

Also, a microphone is used for recording the snoring sounds or comments of the examiner. The examination is started with the patient in a supine position. Later on, different body positions or head rotations can be performed to investigate the influence of different positions during DISE.[59,60] As a sedation target, propofol is highly recommended due to its safety aspects.[30] Hillman et al also showed that UA collapsibility occurs abruptly beyond loss of consciousness within a narrow range of propofol concentration. This change happens nonlinearly with respect to increased propofol concentrations and can be seen in a decrease in entropy or BIS.[58] This is one reason why propofol should be applied by a target-controlled infusion (TCI) pump during DISE. TCI should start with a target concentration of $2.0\,\mu g/mL$ and increase stepwise every 90 s by $0.1\,\mu g/mL$.[34] Three levels of sedation can be defined: light sedation (SE levels > 80%), medium sedation (SE levels between 60 and 80%), and deep sedation (SE dropped below 60%). Sedation should be stopped if SE drops below 50%. If entropy or BIS measuring is not available, clinical examinations as lack of verbal response and starting of snoring can be used as a tool for sedation level of the patient. Also, it is recommended that patients should be monitored postprocedure until complete orientation is restored, and persistent cardio respiratory stability can be ensured. A flexible endoscope is used transnasally and positioned before the procedure begins to get an impression of what happens in the UA during increasing sedation/sleep. In our department, the VOTE classification is used to standardize the grading system.[35] The entire endoscopy should be recorded. As a maneuver, a jaw thrust (Esmarch maneuver) should be performed to its impact on the UA (▶ Table 18.2).

18.5 Analyzing the Results of DISE in Patients with Breathing-Synchronized HNS

▶ Fig. 18.2a, b shows the analysis of our own DISE results in OSA patients with breathing-synchronized HNS who received this examination as a screening tool before surgery. It is remarkable that more than 85% of the implanted patients showed an AP collapse at the soft palate during DISE before surgery. With a responder rate of more than 90%, *even* these patients are perfect candidates for this unique therapy.[61] Due to the fact that all implanted patients have moderate-to-severe sleep apnea, it is known that multilevel collapse is most often detected.[62] So, it is not surprising that many patients also have obstruction at the tongue base (75%). However, even patients with no obstruction at the tongue base and just collapse at the soft palate can be perfect candidates for breathing-synchronized HNS.

Table 18.2 Obstruction patterns during DISE, which are suitable for UAS, and its involved muscle groups, which are responsible for opening the affected anatomic level.

	Suitable obstruction patterns for UAS in DISE	Involved muscle groups for opening	HN fibers	Recommendation for inclusion
Velum	AP, lateral	Palatoglossus muscle	Intrinsic transverse and vertical muscle fibers (T/V)	*Strong*
Orolateral pharyngeal wall	Lateral	Genioglossus and palatoglossus muscles	Main medial branches of HN	*Strong*
Tongue Base	AP	Genioglossus muscle	Main medial branches of HN	*Strong*
Epiglottis	AP, lateral	Geniohyoid muscle	First cervical spine nerve (C1)	*Strong*

Abbreviations: AP, anteroposterior; DISE, drug-induced sleep endoscopy; HN, hypoglossal nerve; UAS, upper airway stimulation.
Note: The HN fibers innervating the different intrinsic and extrinsic tongue muscles, are shown, which need to be involved in the stimulation lead.

18.6 Using DISE as a Titration Tool for Hypoglossal Nerve Stimulation (HNS)

HNS usually is activated first during wakefulness in order to assess thresholds for sensation, functional, and subdiscomfort levels. In selective UAS (Inspire), breathing sensor signals are assessed to secure stimulation synchronized with respiration. In continuous stimulation (ImThera), thresholds have to be detected for each of the six contacts. If titration during sleep is difficult and insufficient in eliminating obstructed breathing, then titration during DISE may be useful. It allows visualizing airway behavior at different stimulation patterns and amplitudes, thus revealing reasons for therapy failure and their treatment. Titration can be done during sleep, gradually increasing the stimulation amplitude or changing other parameters while scoping the pharynx and larynx. We noticed the following findings with selective breathing-synchronized HNS: change of the collapse pattern from AP retropalatal to concentric retropalatal due to weight gain being reversible by weight loss; persistence of a palatal collapse despite strong tongue protrusion being reversible by additional soft palate surgery with or without tonsillectomy; required stimulation amplitudes being higher than subdiscomfort level being reversible by changing further parameters such as frequency or pulse width and thus reducing the amplitude; occurrence of a floppy epiglottis despite strong tongue protrusion being reversible by switching from bipolar to monopolar stimulation, thus widening the electrical field toward C1, activating the geniohyoid muscle.[18] For continuous HNS it may additionally be difficult to differentiate those contacts stabilizing

the airway during wakefulness and sleep in some cases. DISE is able to help recognizing beneficial contacts or combinations of contacts, thus reducing the number of titration nights needed.

References

[1] Strollo PJ, Jr, Soose RJ, Maurer JT, et al. STAR Trial Group. Upper-airway stimulation for obstructive sleep apnea. N Engl J Med. 2014; 370(2):139–149

[2] Heiser C, Maurer JT, Steffen A. Selective upper airway stimulation: German post market study. Sleep. 2016; 39(Supplement):136–137

[3] Heiser C, Maurer JT, Hofauer B, Sommer JU, Seitz A, Steffen A. Outcomes of upper airway stimulation for obstructive sleep apnea in a multicenter german postmarket study. Otolaryngol Head Neck Surg. 2017; 156(2):378–384

[4] Steffen A, Sommer JU, Hofauer B, Maurer JT, Hasselbacher K, Heiser C. Outcome after one year of upper airway stimulation for obstructive sleep apnea in a multicenter German post-market study. Laryngoscope. 2018; 128(2):509–515

[5] Boon M, Huntley C, Steffen A, et al. ADHERE Registry Investigators. Upper airway stimulation for obstructive sleep apnea: results from the ADHERE registry. Otolaryngol Head Neck Surg. 2018; 159(2): 379–385

[6] Woodson BT, Soose RJ, Gillespie MB, et al. STAR Trial Investigators. Three-year outcomes of cranial nerve stimulation for obstructive sleep apnea: the STAR trial. Otolaryngol Head Neck Surg. 2016; 154 (1):181–188

[7] Woodson BT, Strohl KP, Soose RJ, et al. Upper airway stimulation for obstructive sleep apnea: 5-year outcomes. Otolaryngol Head Neck Surg. 2018:194599818762383

[8] Hofauer B, Heiser C. The use of selective upper airway stimulation therapy in Germany. Somnologie (Berl). 2018; 22(2):98–105

[9] Heiser C, Hofauer B. [Hypoglossal nerve stimulation in patients with CPAP failure: Evolution of an alternative treatment for patients with obstructive sleep apnea]. HNO. 2017; 65(2):99–106

[10] Friedman M, Jacobowitz O, Hwang MS, et al. Targeted hypoglossal nerve stimulation for the treatment of obstructive sleep apnea: Six-month results. Laryngoscope. 2016; 126(11):2618–2623

[11] Sommer JU, Hörmann K. Innovative surgery for obstructive sleep apnea: nerve stimulator. Adv Otorhinolaryngol. 2017; 80:116–124

[12] Heiser C, Maurer JT, Steffen A. Functional outcome of tongue motions with selective hypoglossal nerve stimulation in patients with obstructive sleep apnea. Sleep Breath. 2016; 20(2):553–560

[13] Heiser C, Thaler E, Boon M, Soose RJ, Woodson BT. Updates of operative techniques for upper airway stimulation. Laryngoscope. 2016; 126 Suppl 7:S12–S16

[14] Heiser C, Hofauer B, Lozier L, Woodson BT, Stark T. Nerve monitoring-guided selective hypoglossal nerve stimulation in obstructive sleep apnea patients. Laryngoscope. 2016; 126(12):2852–2858

[15] Heiser C, Knopf A, Hofauer B. Surgical anatomy of the hypoglossal nerve: A new classification system for selective upper airway stimulation. Head Neck. 2017; 39(12):2371–2380

[16] Heiser C, Thaler E, Soose RJ, Woodson BT, Boon M. Technical tips during implantation of selective upper airway stimulation. Laryngoscope. 2017

[17] Heiser C, Hofauer B. [Hypoglossal nerve stimulation in patients with CPAP failure: evolution of an alternative treatment for patients with obstructive sleep apnea]. HNO. 2016

[18] Heiser C. Advanced titration to treat a floppy epiglottis in selective upper airway stimulation. Laryngoscope. 2016; 126 Suppl 7:S22–S24

[19] Mwenge GB, Rombaux P, Dury M, Lengelé B, Rodenstein D. Targeted hypoglossal neurostimulation for obstructive sleep apnoea: a 1-year pilot study. Eur Respir J. 2013; 41(2):360–367

[20] Rodenstein D, Rombaux P, Lengele B, Dury M, Mwenge GB. Residual effect of THN hypoglossal stimulation in obstructive sleep apnea: a disease-modifying therapy. Am J Respir Crit Care Med. 2013; 187 (11):1276–1278

[21] Vanderveken OM, Maurer JT, Hohenhorst W, et al. Evaluation of drug-induced sleep endoscopy as a patient selection tool for implanted upper airway stimulation for obstructive sleep apnea. J Clin Sleep Med. 2013; 9(5):433–438

[22] Safiruddin F, Vanderveken OM, de Vries N, et al. Effect of upper-airway stimulation for obstructive sleep apnoea on airway dimensions. Eur Respir J. 2015; 45(1):129–138

[23] Van de Heyning PH, Badr MS, Baskin JZ, et al. Implanted upper airway stimulation device for obstructive sleep apnea. Laryngoscope. 2012; 122(7):1626–1633

[24] Schwartz AR, Barnes M, Hillman D, et al. Acute upper airway responses to hypoglossal nerve stimulation during sleep in obstructive sleep apnea. Am J Respir Crit Care Med. 2012; 185(4):420–426

[25] Kezirian EJ, Boudewyns A, Eisele DW, et al. Electrical stimulation of the hypoglossal nerve in the treatment of obstructive sleep apnea. Sleep Med Rev. 2010; 14(5):299–305

[26] Eastwood PR, Barnes M, Walsh JH, et al. Treating obstructive sleep apnea with hypoglossal nerve stimulation. Sleep (Basel). 2011; 34 (11):1479–1486

[27] Schwartz AR, Bennett ML, Smith PL, et al. Therapeutic electrical stimulation of the hypoglossal nerve in obstructive sleep apnea. Arch Otolaryngol Head Neck Surg. 2001; 127(10):1216–1223

[28] Mu L, Sanders I. Human tongue neuroanatomy: nerve supply and motor endplates. Clin Anat. 2010; 23(7):777–791

[29] Sanders I, Mu L. A three-dimensional atlas of human tongue muscles. Anat Rec (Hoboken). 2013; 296(7):1102–1114

[30] De Vito A, Carrasco Llatas M, Vanni A, et al. European position paper on drug-induced sedation endoscopy (DISE). Sleep Breath. 2014; 18(3): 453–465

[31] Verse T, Dreher A, Heiser C, et al. ENT-specific therapy of obstructive sleep apnoea in adults: a revised version of the previously published German S2e guideline. Sleep Breath. 2016; 20(4):1301–1311

[32] Croft CB, Pringle M. Sleep nasendoscopy: a technique of assessment in snoring and obstructive sleep apnoea. Clin Otolaryngol Allied Sci. 1991; 16(5):504–509

[33] Eastwood PR, Szollosi I, Platt PR, Hillman DR. Comparison of upper airway collapse during general anaesthesia and sleep. Lancet. 2002; 359(9313):1207–1209

[34] Heiser C, Fthenakis P, Hapfelmeier A, et al. Drug-induced sleep endoscopy with target-controlled infusion using propofol and monitored

depth of sedation to determine treatment strategies in obstructive sleep apnea. Sleep Breath. 2017; 21(3):737–744

[35] Kezirian EJ, Hohenhorst W, de Vries N. Drug-induced sleep endoscopy: the VOTE classification. Eur Arch Otorhinolaryngol. 2011; 268 (8):1233–1236

[36] Vicini C, De Vito A, Benazzo M, et al. The nose oropharynx hypopharynx and larynx (NOHL) classification: a new system of diagnostic standardized examination for OSAHS patients. Eur Arch Otorhinolaryngol. 2012; 269(4):1297–1300

[37] Heiser C, Edenharter G, Bas M, Wirth M, Hofauer B. Palatoglossus coupling in selective upper airway stimulation. Laryngoscope. 2017; 127(10):E378–E383

[38] Ferguson KA, Love LL, Ryan CF. Effect of mandibular and tongue protrusion on upper airway size during wakefulness. Am J Respir Crit Care Med. 1997; 155(5):1748–1754

[39] Mortimore IL, Douglas NJ. Palatal muscle EMG response to negative pressure in awake sleep apneic and control subjects. Am J Respir Crit Care Med. 1997; 156(3 Pt 1):867–873

[40] Van de Graaff WB, Gottfried SB, Mitra J, van Lunteren E, Cherniack NS, Strohl KP. Respiratory function of hyoid muscles and hyoid arch. J Appl Physiol. 1984; 57(1):197–204

[41] ElShebiny T, Venkat D, Strohl K, Hans MG, Alonso A, Palomo JM. Hyoid arch displacement with hypoglossal nerve stimulation. Am J Respir Crit Care Med. 2017; 196(6):790–792

[42] Collier CR, Dail CW, Affeldt JE. Mechanics of glossopharyngeal breathing. J Appl Physiol. 1956; 8(6):580–584

[43] Mazza FG, DiMarco AF, Altose MD, Strohl KP. The flow-volume loop during glossopharyngeal breathing. Chest. 1984; 85(5):638–640

[44] Friedman M, Salapatas AM, Bonzelaar LB. Updated Friedman staging system for obstructive sleep apnea. Adv Otorhinolaryngol. 2017; 80: 41–48

[45] Sommer UJ, Heiser C, Gahleitner C, et al. Tonsillectomy with uvulopalatopharyngoplasty in obstructive sleep apnea. Dtsch Arztebl Int. 2016; 113(1–02):1–8

[46] Defalque RJ, Wright AJ. Who invented the "jaw thrust"? Anesthesiology. 2003; 99(6):1463–1464

[47] Eckert DJ, Malhotra A, Lo YL, White DP, Jordan AS. The influence of obstructive sleep apnea and gender on genioglossus activity during rapid eye movement sleep. Chest. 2009; 135(4):957–964

[48] Eckert DJ. Phenotypic approaches to positional therapy for obstructive sleep apnoea. Sleep Med Rev. 2018; 37:175–176

[49] Martins RT, Carberry JC, Eckert DJ. Breath-to-breath reflex modulation of genioglossus muscle activity in obstructive sleep apnea. Sleep Med. 2016; 21:45–46

[50] Zaidi FN, Meadows P, Jacobowitz O, Davidson TM. Tongue anatomy and physiology, the scientific basis for a novel targeted neurostimulation system designed for the treatment of obstructive sleep apnea. Neuromodulation. 2013; 16(4):376–386, discussion 386

[51] Heiser C, Hofauer B. [Stimulation for sleep apnea: targeting the hypoglossal nerve in the treatment of patients with OSA]. HNO. 2018

[52] Takahashi S, Ono T, Ishiwata Y, Kuroda T. Breathing modes, body positions, and suprahyoid muscle activity. J Orthod. 2002; 29(4): 307–313, discussion 279

[53] Zhu Z, Hofauer B, Heiser C. Improving surgical results in complex nerve anatomy during implantation of selective upper airway stimulation. Auris Nasus Larynx. 2018; 45(3):653–656

[54] Heiser C, Thaler E, Soose RJ, Woodson BT, Boon M. Technical tips during implantation of selective upper airway stimulation. Laryngoscope. 2018; 128(3):756–762

[55] Steffen A, Kilic A, Konig IR, Suurna MV, Hofauer B, Heiser C. Tongue motion variability with changes of upper airway stimulation electrode configuration and effects on treatment outcomes. Laryngoscope. 2017

[56] Heiser C, Edenharter GM. Response to "is sedation administration strategy and analysis during drug-induced sedation endoscopy objective and systematic?". Sleep Breath. 2018; 22(1):183–184

[57] Schmidt GN, Bischoff P, Standl T, Hellstern A, Teuber O, Schulte Esch J. Comparative evaluation of the Datex-Ohmeda S/5 Entropy Module and

the Bispectral Index monitor during propofol-remifentanil anesthesia. Anesthesiology. 2004; 101(6):1283–1290

[58] Hillman DR, Walsh JH, Maddison KJ, et al. Evolution of changes in upper airway collapsibility during slow induction of anesthesia with propofol. Anesthesiology. 2009; 111(1):63–71

[59] Safiruddin F, Koutsourelakis I, de Vries N. Analysis of the influence of head rotation during drug-induced sleep endoscopy in obstructive sleep apnea. Laryngoscope. 2014; 124(9).2195–2199

[60] Safiruddin F, Koutsourelakis I, de Vries N. Upper airway collapse during drug induced sleep endoscopy: head rotation in supine position compared with lateral head and trunk position. Eur Arch Otorhinolaryngol. 2015; 272(2):485–488

[61] Heiser C, Knopf A, Bas M, Gahleitner C, Hofauer B. Selective upper airway stimulation for obstructive sleep apnea: a single center clinical experience. Eur Arch Otorhinolaryngol. 2017; 274(3): 1727–1734

[62] Ong AA, Murphey AW, Nguyen SA, et al. Efficacy of upper airway stimulation on collapse patterns observed during drug-induced sedation endoscopy. Otolaryngol Head Neck Surg. 2016; 154(5): 970–977

19 DISE and Treatment with Mandibular Advancement Devices in Obstructive Sleep Apnea Patients

Patty E. Vonk, Madeline J.L. Ravesloot, Olivier M. Vanderveken, Anneclaire V.M.T. Vroegop, and Nico de Vries

Abstract

This chapter focuses on the role of drug-induced sleep endoscopy (DISE) in case treatment with a mandibular advancement device (MAD) is considered. The role of DISE for this indication remains controversial.

Is DISE of added value before commencing MAD treatment to improve treatment success? In this chapter, we discuss the role of DISE and application of various passive maneuvers, simulation bites and a remotely controlled mandibular positioner during DISE in predicting MAD treatment success.

Keywords: dental sleep medicine, DISE, mandibular advancement device (MAD) treatment, oral appliance therapy (OAT), sleep-disordered breathing, obstructive sleep apnea (OSA)

19.1 Introduction

Historically, continuous positive airway pressure (CPAP) is considered the standard therapy for moderate-to-severe obstructive sleep apnea (OSA), but its noncompliance rate is often high due to poor tolerance and low acceptance.[1,2,3] Treatment with oral appliances have been demonstrated to be an effective alternative in patients with mild-to-moderate OSA or in cases of CPAP intolerance or failure. The most commonly used class of oral appliances used for the treatment of sleep-disordered breathing (SDB) are the so-called mandibular advancement devices (MADs). MADs aim at protruding the mandible during sleep, thereby enlarging the collapsible segment of the upper airway (UA). The current recommendation is to use custom-made, titratable MADs.[2,3]

As mentioned before, DISE is a diagnostic tool for upper airway (UA) evaluation in patients with SDB, and in many cases, observations made during drug-induced sleep endoscopy (DISE) alter patient management and optimize the selection for suitable candidates for UA surgery.[4,5,6] However, the role of DISE in predicting treatment outcome of conservative treatment options for OSA, in particular MAD treatment, is more controversial and in most centers not part of daily practice.

19.2 MAD Treatment Success

MAD is commonly used in patients with mild-to-moderate OSA or in case of CPAP failure in moderate and severe diseases. In order to prevent UA obstruction, MADs are designed to advance the mandible in a forward position.

The tongue base, epiglottis and soft palate are protruded, and as a consequence, cross-sectional UA dimensions are increased, reducing snoring and UA collapse.[7] In addition, MADs may also stimulate the musculature of the palate, tongue and pharynx, resulting in decreased UA resistance.[8]

Previous studies have shown that in patients with OSA, MADs are successful in a substantial proportion of patients. Differences in treatment success of MAD are likely to be related to the variation in definitions of treatment success. Overall, a complete therapeutic response (treatment apnea–hypopnea index [AHI] < 5 events/h) is seen in 29 to 71% with an average of 48%. In most studies, OSA patients with mild-to-moderate OSA are included.[3] In severe OSA patients, treatment success is lower. Walker-Engström et al compared the effect of a MAD with a mandibular advancement of 50% and 75%. MAD was successful in reducing AHI < 5 events/h in 31% and 52%, respectively.[9] Hoekema et al found a higher success rate of 69%, but used a different definition of treatment success, namely, a treatment AHI < 5 events/h or a reduction in AHI of at least 50% from baseline value to a value of < 20 events/h and the absence of OSA-related symptoms.[10]

The residual OSA might be explained by the difficult identification of suitable patients for MAD and by the lack of predictive factors in predicting treatment outcome and success. Predictors including body mass index (BMI), AHI, age, gender, cephalometric findings and polysomnographic outcomes have been variously associated with treatment outcome with oral appliance therapy (OAT).[11] However, not only is a patient's baseline UA anatomy/collapsibility important but the nonanatomic trait loop gain also seems to play a major role in predicting treatment success.[12] The value of observations made during DISE vary among studies, but several studies have shown that MADs are less effective in cases of a complete concentric collapse at the level of the palate (CCCp).[13,14]

19.3 DISE as a Screening Tool for MAD Treatment

Currently, the question that has arisen is if DISE is of added value before commencing MAD treatment to improve treatment success. The considerations are as follows: with MAD, "one gets what one pays for," and the most effective MADs with the best fit are expensive. The production and titration of a MAD with, at times, a repeated sleep study is an expensive and lengthy process. In case the MAD does not provide the desired effect, it cannot be reused in another patient. The alternative would be to perform DISE first and mimic the effect of a MAD by performing a jaw thrust, using a simulation bite, or a remotely controlled mandibular positioner (RCMP), and only start with the MAD production and fitting process in case of a positive effect of mandibular protrusion during DISE. Although the complications and side effects of DISE are negligible, this approach involves extra time and money as well. Therefore, two situations need to be distinguished: MAD treatment as the only therapeutic option under consideration; second, where multiple treatment options, including both conservative and surgical, are feasible, whereby choice of treatment is, amongst others, dependent on DISE findings.

One of the advantages of DISE is that it allows the physician to perform different passive maneuvers with reassessment of UA patency after each maneuver. The maneuvers relevant for this chapter aim to mimic the effect and prospectively predict treatment success of a MAD. Two maneuvers have been described: chin-lift and jaw thrust (e.g., Esmarch maneuver). A chin-lift is a manual closure of the mouth (▶ Fig. 19.1), while a jaw thrust is a gentle advancement of the mandible up to approximately 5 mm (▶ Fig. 19.2).[15]

Besides the fact that a MAD causes advancement of the mandible, it is clear that a specific MAD also comes with a given thickness, causing vertical opening (VO) of the mouth. Vroegop et al evaluated the clinical relevance of VO and found that VO of the mouth is another variable that must be taken into consideration, since VO tends to have an adverse effect on the cross-sectional area of the tongue base. The maneuver of mouth closure and opening can be easily added to the DISE procedure.[16]

As previously mentioned, the use of DISE before initiation of MAD is controversial and the predictive value of DISE for MAD treatment success varies among studies. Eichler et al evaluated to what extent performing DISE, including jaw thrust, resulted in changes in treatment recommendations as compared to the basic ENT clinical examination. It was concluded that the effect of mandibular advancement on UA patency could be evaluated during DISE, resulting in changes in treatment recommendations in the majority of patients. One of the recommendations with the highest rate of change was MAD, suggesting DISE as a relevant examination to be included in the screening of suitable candidates for MAD treatment.[17] Furthermore, Johal et al found a good correlation between jaw thrust and treatment success rate.[18,19] These results are supported by Huntley et al. They concluded that patients with increased airway dimensions at the level of the velum and/or oropharynx with jaw thrust during DISE may benefit most from MAD treatment and suggested that the use of DISE can be helpful in optimizing treatment outcome.[20]

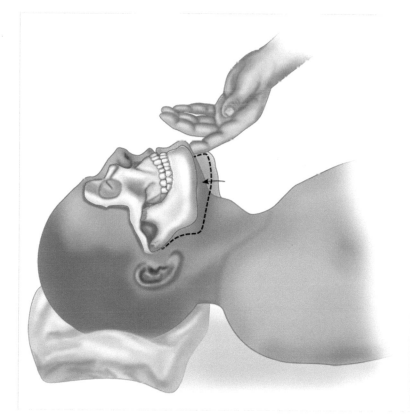

Fig. 19.1 Chin-lift, a manual closure of the mouth.

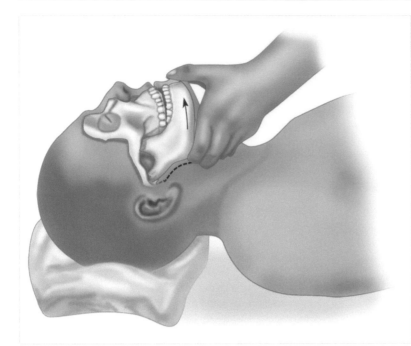

Fig. 19.2 Jaw thrust, or Esmarch maneuver, a gentle advancement of the mandible by up to approximately 5 mm.

In contrast, Vanderveken et al and Vroegop et al have been questioning the correlation between the effect of chin-lift during DISE and treatment success of MAD and suggested the use of a simulation bite in a reproducible maximal comfortable protrusion (MCP) during DISE, which tended to better predict response to MAD.[21,22]

By performing jaw thrust, the mandible is actively protruded, with the aim to mimic the protrusive position of the mandible achieved with a MAD.[23] It is clear that this maneuver is not similar to the real-life effect of a MAD. First, as stated before, it does not take the thickness of a MAD into account and therefore does not take the effect of VO of the mouth into consideration. Second, a MAD is usually set at 60 to 75% of maximum protrusion. When applying jaw thrust, is it difficult to estimate the desired degree of mandible advancement. The latter two may contribute to the variation in the predictive value of manually performed jaw thrust in response to MAD treatment.

19.4 Thermoplastic Appliances

In 2008 Vanderveken et al evaluated the efficacy of a thermoplastic appliance compared to a classic custom-made MAD. They evaluated whether a thermoplastic appliance could be used as a screening tool in predicting MAD success. They concluded that a custom-made MAD was more effective than a thermoplastic monobloc device, and that the thermoplastic MAD evaluated in that particular study could not be recommended as a screening method for treatment success. A significant percentage (73%) of all

compliance failures in the thermoplastic appliance group was due to a lack of retention of the appliance.[24]

19.5 Simulation Bite and a Remotely Controlled Mandibular Positioner

The accuracy of the jaw thrust and chin-lift maneuvers has been questioned, and more accurate alternatives suggested in literature are a simulation bite and a RCMP.[21,22,25,26] A simulation bite can be custom-made for each individual patient, with a dedicated registration fork and the upper arch covered with a bite-registration material, placed against the upper tooth arch (▸ Fig. 19.3). After curing, the patient is instructed to protrude the mandible forward toward the MCP. These measurements are then repeated three times, measured, and averaged. This averaged position is then recorded with the lower arch of the fork, using the same bite-registration material, resulting in the simulation bite in MCP.[16]

A RCMP consists of impression trays filled with a rigid impression material, mimicking the MAD positioned in the mouth of the patient, attached to a positioner, which progressively protrudes the mandible through a controller located in a patient monitoring room.[25,27] It has been shown that the use of RCMP during sleep studies predicts therapeutic success with MADs in patients with OSA.[26]

The use of a simulation bite provides a reliable and reproducible mandibular position, taking into account

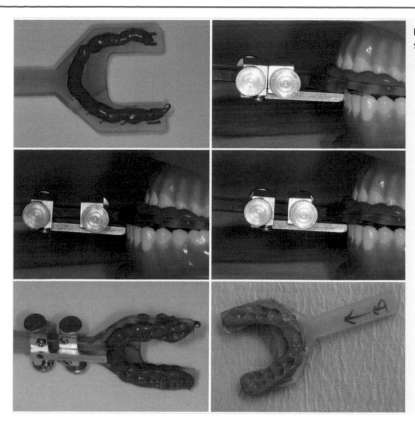

Fig. 19.3 Overview of a custom-made simulation bite.

the given thickness of a particular MAD, whereas each oral appliance inherently causes a certain amount of VO of the mouth, as noted previously. An additional advantage of the use of simulation bites and similar devices is that disturbing stimuli, potentially provoking awakening, as with the jaw thrust and chin-lift maneuvers, can be avoided.

19.6 Conclusions

The use of DISE before initiation of MAD is still controversial and the predictive value of DISE for MAD treatment success varies among studies. Nevertheless, custom-made simulation bites have proven to be successful in predicting therapeutic success with MADs in patients with OSA.[26] The use of a simulation bite seems to be more predictive compared to the jaw thrust, and the use of these devices should be outweighed against the additional costs and effort accompanied by a dental examination and construction of a simulation bite before DISE. These factors can be dependent of local infrastructure, policy and reimbursement criteria and are not yet part of common practice. Before DISE will be accepted as a generally used screening tool for patient selection for MAD, there is a need for a relative cheap, quick and easy-to-use system to mimic the effect of a MAD during DISE, which could also be of interest in research settings.

References

[1] Rotenberg BW, Vicini C, Pang EB, Pang KP. Reconsidering first-line treatment for obstructive sleep apnea: a systematic review of the literature. J Otolaryngol Head Neck Surg. 2016; 45:23

[2] Marklund M, Verbraecken J, Randerath W. Non-CPAP therapies in obstructive sleep apnoea: mandibular advancement device therapy. Eur Respir J. 2012; 39(5):1241–1247

[3] Sutherland K, Vanderveken OM, Tsuda H, et al. Oral appliance treatment for obstructive sleep apnea: an update. J Clin Sleep Med. 2014; 10(2):215–227

[4] Huntley C, Chou D, Doghramji K, Boon M. Preoperative drug induced sleep endoscopy improves the surgical approach to treatment of obstructive sleep apnea. Ann Otol Rhinol Laryngol. 2017; 126(6):478–482

[5] Certal VF, Pratas R, Guimarães L, et al. Awake examination versus DISE for surgical decision making in patients with OSA: a systematic review. Laryngoscope. 2016; 126(3):768–774

[6] Vanderveken OM, Maurer JT, Hohenhorst W, et al. Evaluation of drug-induced sleep endoscopy as a patient selection tool for implanted upper airway stimulation for obstructive sleep apnea. J Clin Sleep Med. 2013; 9(5):433–438

[7] Tsuiki S, Lowe AA, Almeida FR, Kawahata N, Fleetham JA. Effects of mandibular advancement on airway curvature and obstructive sleep apnoea severity. Eur Respir J. 2004; 23(2):263–268

[8] Chan AS, Lee RW, Cistulli PA. Dental appliance treatment for obstructive sleep apnea. Chest. 2007; 132(2):693–699

[9] Walker-Engström M-L, Ringqvist I, Vestling O, Wilhelmsson B, Tegelberg A. A prospective randomized study comparing two different degrees of mandibular advancement with a dental appliance in treatment of severe obstructive sleep apnea. Sleep Breath. 2003; 7 (3):119–130

[10] Hoekema A, Stegenga B, Wijkstra PJ, van der Hoeven JH, Meinesz AF, de Bont LG. Obstructive sleep apnea therapy. J Dent Res. 2008; 87(9): 882–887

[11] Sutherland K, Takaya H, Qian J, Petocz P, Ng AT, Cistulli PA. Oral appliance treatment response and polysomnographic phenotypes of obstructive sleep apnea. J Clin Sleep Med. 2015; 11(8):861–868

[12] Edwards BA, Andara C, Landry S, et al. Upper-airway collapsibility and loop gain predict the response to oral appliance therapy in patients with obstructive sleep apnea. Am J Respir Crit Care Med. 2016; 194(11):1413–1422

[13] Dieltjens M, Wouters K, Verbruggen A, et al. Drug-induced sedation endoscopy (DISE) findings correlate with treatment outcome in OSA patients treated with oral appliance therapy in a fixed mandibular protrusion. Am J Respir Crit Care Med. 2015; 191:A2474

[14] Op de Beeck S, Dieltjens M, Verbruggen AE, et al. Phenotypic labeling using drug-induced sleep endoscopy improves patient selection for mandibular advancement device outcome. American journal of respiratory and critical care medicine

[15] Hohenhorst W, Ravesloot M, Kezirian E, De Vries N. Drug-induced sleep endoscopy in adults with sleep-disordered breathing: technique and the VOTE classification system. Oper Tech Otolaryngol–Head Neck Surg. 2012; 23(1):11–18

[16] Vroegop AV, Vanderveken OM, Van de Heyning PH, Braem MJ. Effects of vertical opening on pharyngeal dimensions in patients with obstructive sleep apnoea. Sleep Med. 2012; 13(3):314–316

[17] Eichler C, Sommer JU, Stuck BA, Hörmann K, Maurer JT. Does drug-induced sleep endoscopy change the treatment concept of patients with snoring and obstructive sleep apnea? Sleep Breath. 2013; 17(1):63–68

[18] Johal A, Battagel JM, Kotecha BT. Sleep nasendoscopy: a diagnostic tool for predicting treatment success with mandibular advancement splints in obstructive sleep apnoea. Eur J Orthod. 2005; 27(6):607–614

[19] Johal A, Hector MP, Battagel JM, Kotecha BT. Impact of sleep nasendoscopy on the outcome of mandibular advancement splint therapy in subjects with sleep-related breathing disorders. J Laryngol Otol. 2007; 121(7):668–675

[20] Huntley C, Cooper J, Stiles M, Grewal R, Boon M. Predicting success of oral appliance therapy in treating obstructive sleep apnea using drug-induced sleep endoscopy. J Clin Sleep Med. 2018; 14(8):1333–1337

[21] Vroegop AV, Vanderveken OM, Dieltjens M, et al. Sleep endoscopy with simulation bite for prediction of oral appliance treatment outcome. J Sleep Res. 2013; 22(3):348–355

[22] Vanderveken OM, Vroegop AV, Van de Heyning PH, Braem MJ. Drug-induced sleep endoscopy completed with a simulation bite approach for the prediction of the outcome of treatment of obstructive sleep apnea with mandibular repositioning appliances. Oper Tech Otolaryngol–Head Neck Surg. 2011; 22(2):175–182

[23] Vanderveken OM. Drug-induced sleep endoscopy (DISE) for non-CPAP treatment selection in patients with sleep-disordered breathing. Sleep Breath. 2013; 17(1):13–14

[24] Vanderveken OM, Devolder A, Marklund M, et al. Comparison of a custom-made and a thermoplastic oral appliance for the treatment of mild sleep apnea. Am J Respir Crit Care Med. 2008; 178(2):197–202

[25] Kastoer C, Dieltjens M, Oorts E, et al. The use of remotely controlled mandibular positioner as a predictive screening tool for mandibular advancement device therapy in patients with obstructive sleep apnea through single-night progressive titration of the mandible: a systematic review. J Clin Sleep Med. 2016; 12(10):1411–1421

[26] Tsai WH, Vazquez JC, Oshima T, et al. Remotely controlled mandibular positioner predicts efficacy of oral appliances in sleep apnea. Am J Respir Crit Care Med. 2004; 170(4):366–370

[27] Remmers JE, Topor Z, Grosse J, et al. A feedback-controlled mandibular positioner identifies individuals with sleep apnea who will respond to oral appliance therapy. J Clin Sleep Med. 2017; 13(7):871–880

20 The Use of DISE to Determine Candidates for Upper Airway Stimulation

Adrian A. Ong and M. Boyd Gillespie

Abstract

Obstructive sleep apnea (OSA) is a complex medical condition resulting from loss of neuromuscular tone of the upper airway (UA) and subsequent airflow obstruction. Upper airway stimulation (UAS) is the first surgical intervention to directly address the pathophysiology of increased airway collapsibility during sleep. UAS acts by stimulating the hypoglossal nerve (HN), and activating the genioglossus muscle and associated airway dilators. Direct coupling of the base of tongue to the soft palate via the palatoglossus muscle results in airway dilation at multiple levels of the UA. Drug-induced sleep endoscopy (DISE) is an essential component of the preoperative evaluation of UAS, as complete concentric collapse of the soft palate is a contraindication to UAS implantation. Patients who do not qualify for UAS due to complete concentric collapse of the soft palate on DISE may benefit from variations of uvulopalatopharyngoplasty (UPPP) that alters the collapse pattern at the soft palate, possibly allowing patients to become eligible for UAS implantation at a later date.

Keywords: drug-induced sedation endoscopy, drug-induced sleep endoscopy, upper airway stimulation, hypoglossal nerve stimulation, obstructive sleep apnea, sleep-disordered breathing

20.1 Introduction

The gold standard treatment of obstructive sleep apnea (OSA) continues to be continuous positive airway pressure (CPAP). Unfortunately, up to 50% of patients are unable to tolerate CPAP and use it less than the recommended minimum of 4 hours per night.[1] In these patients, surgical management of OSA is an option; however, patients may be cautious in pursuing these procedures due to the high morbidity and inconsistent symptom improvement.[2] Recently, upper airway stimulation (UAS) was introduced as a novel implantable device which decreases the collapsibility of the UA via stimulation of the hypoglossal nerve (HN).[3] During the clinical trial which validated the safety and efficacy of UAS, drug-induced sleep endoscopy (DISE) was utilized during the preoperative evaluation in order to better select patients likely to respond to UAS. This chapter focuses on UAS as a therapeutic modality, role of DISE in determining candidacy for UAS, and clinical results to date.

20.2 Upper Airway Stimulation (UAS)

20.2.1 History of UAS

UAS was conceptualized as a treatment based on research which demonstrated that a predominant pathophysiology of OSA is the loss of neuromuscular tone during sleep, resulting in upper airway (UA) collapse and airflow obstruction.[4] Specifically, both sleep onset and the hypoxia associated with OSA are associated with loss of genioglossal activity.[5,6] This led to the notion that neural stimulation could be a possible treatment for OSA. Animal studies showed that stimulation of the HN was just as effective as CPAP in reversing inspiratory airflow limitation, and concluded that HN stimulation could be a treatment option for OSA.[7] This ultimately resulted in a pilot human study of HN stimulation which showed improvement in inspiratory airflow with manual stimulation during obstructed inspiration, and led to the development of an implantable UAS device.[8]

20.2.2 UAS Components

The UAS system (Inspire Medical, Maple Grove MN) is an implantable device, which is intended for the treatment of moderate-to-severe OSA, and stimulates the HN during inspiration. ▶ Fig. 20.1 shows the configuration of the UAS device. It consists of multiple components, including an implantable pulse generator (IPG), sensory lead, and stimulation lead as well as a physician and patient programmer.

Sensing Lead

The sensing lead is a pressure transducer which detects the respiratory cycle. It is placed between the internal and external intercostal muscles. The pressure waveform is transmitted to the IPG. The implant is typically placed on the right lateral chest to avoid cardiac artifact and confusion with cardiac pacemakers which are routinely placed on the left upper chest wall.

Implantable Pulse Generator

The IPG contains the programming software and battery and is linked to the sensing and stimulation leads. The programming software directs the synchronization of HN stimulation and inspiration. The battery is expected to last approximately 10 years. The IPG communicates with

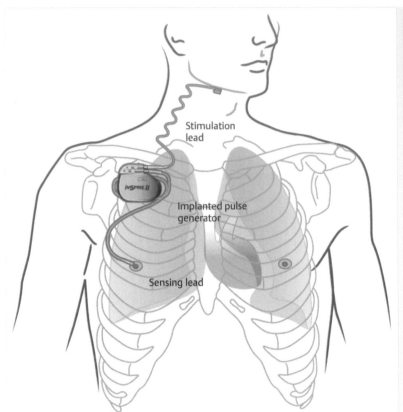

Fig. 20.1 Configuration of the UAS system (Inspire Medical Systems, Minneapolis, MN). Abbreviation: UAS, upper airway stimulation. Reproduced, with permission, from Van de Heyning PH, Badr MS, Baskin JZ, et al. Implanted upper airway stimulation device for obstructive sleep apnea. Laryngoscope. 2012;122(7):1626–1633.

the physician programmer, which regulates the various programming modes, and patient programmer, which has on/off capability and limited programming ability.

Stimulation Lead

The stimulation lead consists of three electrodes on a flexible cuff positioned around the HN. The electrodes can be configured for optimal stimulation of the HN, and thus tongue protrusion to open the pharyngeal airway.

Physician Programmer

The physician programmer allows noninvasive interrogation and programming of the IPG. A telemetry head communicates with the IPG through the skin via short-range radiofrequency telemetry and wirelessly withthe physician programmer. The physician programmer can perform limited self-tests, observe respiratory waveforms, calibrate stimulation modes, modify stimulation parameter values, and record waveforms and patient programmed settings.

Patient Programmer

The patient programmer is an external remote and allows the patient to activate the UAS device prior to

sleep. It has the following functionalities: on/off capability, temporary suspension of therapy, and adjustment of stimulation amplitude (within the physician preselected limit). It also has the ability to check the status of the IPG battery.

20.2.3 Mechanism of UAS

The HN innervates all the intrinsic and extrinsic muscles of the tongue, except the palatoglossus, which is innervated by the vagus nerve. During UAS placement, the stimulating lead is placed in such a way that the primary tongue protrusors (i.e., genioglossus muscle) are stimulated when UAS is activated. With activation of the genioglossus musculature, anterior tongue motion occurs with dilation of the pharyngeal airway. Despite primarily affecting the oropharynx at the level of the tongue base, UAS activation provides a secondary effect of enlarging the UA at the level of the soft palate, primarily in the anteroposterior (AP) direction.[9] This is thought to be due to a mechanical linkage between the tongue base and the soft palate via the palatoglossus muscle. When UAS is activated, tongue protrusion leads to anterior pull on the palatoglossal muscle and movement of the soft palate anteriorly, which positively affects multilevel UA obstruction.

20.2.4 Selection Criteria for UAS

UAS is intended for patients 22 years of age or older with moderate-to-severe OSA who fail or are intolerant to CPAP therapy. Patients undergo a preoperative evaluation, including sleep medicine consultation, surgical consultation, and DISE. During the sleep medicine consultation, a basic history and physical is performed. Ideally, a patient seeking UAS has a body mass index (BMI) ≤ 35 (ideally ≤ 32). Polysomnography (PSG) is obtained to ruleout non-OSA sleep disorders, and to diagnose moderate-to-severe OSA (apnea–hypopnea index [AHI] between 15 events/hour and 65 events/hour). Important contraindications of this therapy are listed in ▶ Table 20.1. During surgical consultation, patients undergo examination while awake with rigid and/or flexible endoscopes to assess for anatomic factors that are considered unfavorable for UAS implantation (▶ Table 20.2). Finally, DISE is performed to rule out the presence of complete concentric collapse of the soft palate (▶ Fig. 20.2). The requirement to use DISE to determine UAS candidacy is based on prior work which showed that patients without complete concentric collapse of the soft palate on DISE had superior outcomes: 81% (13/16 patients) response rate versus 0% (0/5 patients), based on the definition of clinical response of $\geq 50\%$ or more decrease in AHI and postoperative AHI of less than 20 events/hour (▶ Fig. 20.3).[10] The finding of complete concentric collapse suggest that the soft palate collapse in these individuals is not coupled to tongue base collapse and is therefore a contraindication to UAS placement.

20.2.5 Outcomes of UAS

A prospective, multicenter cohort study of 126 patients who fulfilled the selection criteria for UAS implantation was performed to determine the effectiveness of UAS therapy in reducing OSA severity and improving patient-reported outcome measures.[3] The initial results of UAS therapy showed a significant decrease in median AHI from 29.3 events/hour preoperatively to 9.0 events/hour at 12 months postoperatively. This improvement in AHI was sustained at 60 months with a median AHI of 6.2

Table 20.1 Contraindications for use of UAS therapy

Central + mixed apneas > 25% of the total AHI
Any anatomic finding that would compromise the performance of UAS, such as presence of complete concentric collapse of the soft palate
Any condition or procedure that has compromised the neurological control of UA
Patients who are unable or do not have the necessary assistance to operate the sleep remote
Patients who are pregnant or plan to become pregnant
Patients with an implantable device that could experience unintended interaction with the Inspire system
Patients who require MRI

Abbreviations: AHI, apnea–hypopnea index; UA, upper airway; UAS, upper airway stimulation; MRI, magnetic resonance imaging.

Table 20.2 Anatomic findings considered unfavorable for UAS therapy

Nasal cavity	Severe degree of nasal obstruction, and unresponsiveness to pharmacologic treatments, due to conditions such as nasal polyps, nasal valve collapse, prior history of nasal surgery or trauma, etc.
Nasopharynx	Large obstructing adenoid tissue
Velopharynx	Large edematous soft palate
Oropharynx	Large obstructing tonsils (size 3 or 4)
Supraglottis	Laryngomalacia or cyst/mass involving the vallecula/epiglottis with > 75% obstruction at the level of epiglottis
Glottis	Vocal cord polyps causing > 75% obstruction at level of vocal cords, bilateral vocal cord paralysis, and severely edematous and floppy arytenoids with > 75% obstruction at the level of vocal cords
Subglottis	Severe subglottic stenosis

Abbreviation: UAS, upper airway stimulation.

events/hour.[11] In addition, patients had significant improvement in self-reported sleepiness, as measured by the Epworth Sleepiness Scale, improving from a baseline median score of 11 to a median score of 6 at both the 12-month and 60-month mark. These studies concluded that UAS therapy provides long-term, clinically significant improvements in both subjective and objective measures of sleep-disordered breathing (SDB) in this select patient population.

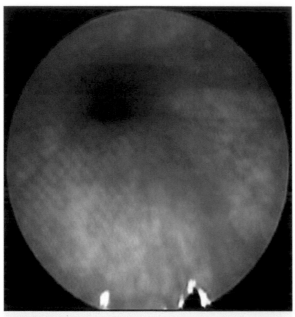

Fig. 20.2 Example of complete concentric collapse of the palate on DISE.

20.3 Clinical History and Data

20.3.1 DISE for UAS Candidacy

Technique

DISE is a standard procedure utilized during the preoperative evaluation for patients seeking UAS for treatment of OSA.[3] DISE is performed with a multidisciplinary team consisting of the otolaryngologist, anesthesiologist, and nursing staff. Monitoring devices, including pulse oximetry, blood pressure, and electrocardiogram, are used during the duration of the procedure. Either a high-resolution flexible nasopharyngoscope or pediatric flexible bronchoscope, with a high-resolution video monitor for observation, is utilized for the study. The capability to digitally record the study for review is optimal.

Prior to DISE, the patient receives a nasal decongestant as well as glycopyrrolate or atropine to decrease the amount of oropharyngeal secretions. These allow for safe and clear viewing when introducing the nasopharyngoscope. Sedation is induced and maintained using IV administration of propofol and/or midazolam, and titrated either by target controlled infusion (TCI) or light sedation where the patient is unarousable to verbal stimulation. Once the patient is no longer responsive to verbal stimuli and begins to snore and/or have mild desaturations, the room lights are dimmed and scope is inserted. The duration of the procedure averages 10 to 15 minutes.

Scoring

DISE is a qualitative and subjective assessment of airway collapse during simulated sleep. The velum,

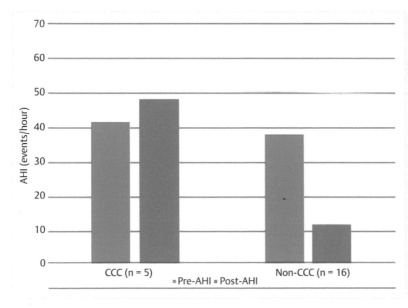

Fig. 20.3 Effect of upper airway stimulation on apnea–hypopnea index in patients with and without complete concentric collapse of the palate. Data from Vanderveken OM, Maurer JT, Hohenhorst W et al. Evaluation of drug-induced sleep endoscopy as a patient selection tool for implanted upper airway stimulation for obstructive sleep apnea. *J Clin Sleep Med* 2013; 9:433–438. Abbreviations: AHI, apnea–hypopnea index; UAS, upper airway stimulation.

Table 20.3 VOTE classification

Structure	Degree of obstruction[a]	Configuration[c]		
		AP	Lateral	Concentric
Velum				
Oropharynx[b]				
Tongue base				
Epiglottis				

Abbreviations: AP, anteroposterior; VOTE, velum, oropharynx, tongue base, and epiglottis.
Data from Kezirian EJ, Hohenhorst W, de Vries N. Drug-induced sleep endoscopy: the VOTE classification. Eur Arch Otorhinolaryngol 2011; 268:1233–1236.
Shaded boxes reflect the fact that a specific structure-configuration cannot be seen.
[a] Degree of obstruction has one number for each structure: 0, No obstruction (no vibration); 1, Partial obstruction (vibration); 2, complete obstruction (collapse); X, Not visualized.
[b] Oropharynx obstruction can be distinguished as related to the tonsils or including the lateral walls, with or without a tonsillar component.
[c] Configuration noted for structures with degree of obstruction greater than zero.

oropharynx, tongue base and epiglottis (VOTE) classification (▶ Table 20.3) is the most commonly used scoring system providing an assessment of the degree and configuration of airway narrowing at four locations of the UA: velum (V), oropharynx lateral walls (O), tongue base (T), and epiglottis (E). At each location, the degree of collapse can be graded as none, partial (vibration, 50–75% narrowing, reduced airflow), or complete (obstruction, >75% narrowing, markedly reduced or absent airflow), while the direction is described as anteroposterior, lateral, or circumferential.[17] As stated prior, the finding of complete concentric collapse of the soft palate is a contraindication to UAS implantation as determined by an earlier feasibility study.

Validity and Reliability of DISE Results for UAS

Although DISE allows direct visualization of the UA during a state that mimics sleep, it is not a perfect depiction of natural sleep. In the case of propofol sedation, prior studies demonstrate a decrease in neuromuscular activity of the genioglossus muscle, which is similar to that observed during nonrapid eye movement sleep, and that low doses did not produce significant changes in AHI or oxygen saturations compared to natural sleep.[13,14] Thus, propofol is considered a good anesthetic choice, allowing for both control of sedation depth and producing a state similar to natural sleep.

Test-retest reliability assesses the similarity of results of distinct examinations in the same patient, and DISE has been shown to have moderate to substantial test-retest reliability.[15] On the other hand, interrater reliability

tests the degree of similarity of agreement between different reviewers. In one study, DISE appears to have moderate to substantial interrater reliability between two experienced surgeons, and in another, interrater reliability was higher amongst experienced surgeons compared to nonexperienced surgeons.[16,17] These results affirm the reliability of DISE as a reliable evaluation tool despite variations in UA collapse patterns among a large cohort of patients.[18] In that particular study, 393 of 1249 patients, or 31%, had complete concentric collapse of the palate, which would preclude UAS implantation. Interrater reliability for complete concentric collapse of the palate on DISE has been evaluated amongst experienced surgeons, and ranged from moderate to substantial.[19] However, in that same study, there was generally poor agreement in determining eligibility for UAS implantation based on DISE. Reasons for not recommending UAS despite absence of complete concentric collapse of the soft palate were not evaluated, although the authors hypothesized that other patterns of obstruction may have been considered to compromise the efficacy of UAS. The variability in recommending UAS therapy based on DISE reinforces the notion that DISE is still a subjective examination. Further training and standardization are needed for more consistent results when it comes to determining UAS candidacy based on DISE results.

20.3.2 Improving UAS Efficacy Using DISE

Although complete concentric collapse of the palate is the only DISE finding which excludes patients from UAS implantation currently, additional studies have evaluated other DISE results in an attempt to improve therapy success. One study assessed the DISE results of patients enrolled in the original prospective, multicenter cohort study and its impact on UAS response rates.[20] This cohort consisted of patients who did not have complete concentric collapse of the palate during preoperative evaluation and underwent implantation after meeting inclusion criteria. They found that patients with increased UA collapsibility, determined by a higher VOTE score, were more likely to be nonresponders to UAS. In addition, those with incomplete response to UAS were more likely to have complete collapse at the level of the soft palate and/or the epiglottis. The authors suggested that based on these findings, there may be a select group of patients who may benefit from a staged surgical approach with uvulopalatopharyngoplasty (UPPP) first followed by UAS implantation.

The effect of UPPP on complete concentric collapse of the palate has also been evaluated.[21] In this study, 15 patients with known complete concentric collapse of the palate were enrolled and underwent tonsillectomy and UPPP. After 3 months, patients underwent repeat DISE: one patient had persistent complete concentric collapse of the palate, 13 had anteroposterior collapse of the palate (nine partial, four complete), and one had no collapse at the palate. These findings suggest that tonsillectomy and UPPP can be offered to change the collapse pattern at the level of the palate for those seeking UAS and found to have complete concentric collapse of the palate, thereby making these patients eligible for UAS implantation.

20.4 Conclusions

UAS is a novel procedure for the treatment of OSA which is effective in carefully selected patients who have failed CPAP therapy. It functions by addressing the underlying pathophysiology of OSA, which is loss of neuromuscular tone of the UA musculature during sleep. Stimulation of the HN improves airflow by opening of the UA at both the base of tongue and soft palate. DISE continues to be a rapid, safe tool in determining candidacy for UAS: complete concentric collapse of the palate is a contraindication to UAS implantation, and there is moderate to substantial agreement among experienced users in their ability to identify this finding. Those who have complete concentric collapse of the palate may benefit from a staged procedure prior to UAS implantation, including UPPP, to alter the collapse pattern seen in DISE. Further prospective and randomized clinical trials are needed to determine additional criteria, such as combinations of collapse patterns which are seen in DISE, in order to improve UAS efficacy.

References

[1] Weaver TE, Grunstein RR. Adherence to continuous positive airway pressure therapy: the challenge to effective treatment. Proc Am Thorac Soc. 2008; 5(2):173–178

[2] Lin HC, Friedman M, Chang HW, Gurpinar B. The efficacy of multilevel surgery of the upper airway in adults with obstructive sleep apnea/hypopnea syndrome. Laryngoscope. 2008; 118(5):902–908

[3] Strollo PJJr, Soose RJ, Maurer JT, et al. STAR Trial Group. Upper-airway stimulation for obstructive sleep apnea. N Engl J Med. 2014; 370(2):139–149

[4] Remmers JE, DeGroot WJ, Sauerland EK, Anch AM. Pathogenesis of upper airway occlusion during sleep. J Appl Physiol. 1978; 44(6):931–938

[5] Kimura H, Niijima M, Edo H, Tatsumi K, Honda Y, Kuriyama T. The effect of hypoxic depression on genioglossal muscle activity in healthy subjects and obstructive sleep apnea patients. Sleep. 1993; 16(8) Suppl:S135–S136

[6] Mezzanotte WS, Tangel DJ, White DP. Influence of sleep onset on upper-airway muscle activity in apnea patients versus normal controls. Am J Respir Crit Care Med. 1996; 153(6 Pt 1):1880–1887

[7] Bellemare F, Pecchiari M, Bandini M, Sawan M, D'Angelo E. Reversibility of airflow obstruction by hypoglossus nerve stimulation in anesthetized rabbits. Am J Respir Crit Care Med. 2005; 172(5):606–612

[8] Eisele DW, Smith PL, Alam DS, Schwartz AR. Direct hypoglossal nerve stimulation in obstructive sleep apnea. Arch Otolaryngol Head Neck Surg. 1997; 123(1):57–61

[9] Safiruddin F, Vanderveken OM, de Vries N, et al. Effect of upper-airway stimulation for obstructive sleep apnoea on airway dimensions. Eur Respir J. 2015; 45(1):129–138

[10] Vanderveken OM, Maurer JT, Hohenhorst W, et al. Evaluation of drug-induced sleep endoscopy as a patient selection tool for implanted upper airway stimulation for obstructive sleep apnea. J Clin Sleep Med. 2013; 9(5):433–438

[11] Woodson BT, Strohl KP, Soose RJ, et al. Upper airway stimulation for obstructive sleep apnea: 5-year outcomes. Otolaryngol Head Neck Surg. 2018; 159(1):194–202

[12] Kezirian EJ, Hohenhorst W, de Vries N. Drug-induced sleep endoscopy: the VOTE classification. Eur Arch Otorhinolaryngol. 2011; 268(8):1233–1236

[13] Hillman DR, Walsh JH, Maddison KJ, et al. Evolution of changes in upper airway collapsibility during slow induction of anesthesia with propofol. Anesthesiology. 2009; 111(1):63–71

[14] Rabelo FA, Braga A, Küpper DS, et al. Propofol-induced sleep: polysomnographic evaluation of patients with obstructive sleep apnea and controls. Otolaryngol Head Neck Surg. 2010; 142(2):218–224

[15] Rodriguez-Bruno K, Goldberg AN, McCulloch CE, Kezirian EJ. Test-retest reliability of drug-induced sleep endoscopy. Otolaryngol Head Neck Surg. 2009; 140(5):646–651

[16] Kezirian EJ, White DP, Malhotra A, Ma W, McCulloch CE, Goldberg AN. Interrater reliability of drug induced sleep endoscopy. Arch Otolaryngol Head Neck Surg. 2010; 136(4):393–397

[17] Vroegop AV, Vanderveken OM, Wouters K, et al. Observer variation in drug-induced sleep endoscopy: experienced versus nonexperienced ear, nose, and throat surgeons. Sleep (Basel). 2013; 36(6):947–953

[18] Vroegop AV, Vanderveken OM, Boudewyns AN, et al. Drug-induced sleep endoscopy in sleep-disordered breathing: report on 1,249 cases. Laryngoscope. 2014; 124(3):797–802

[19] Ong AA, Ayers CM, Kezirian EJ, et al. Application of drug-induced sleep endoscopy in patients treated with upper airway stimulation therapy. World J Otorhinolaryngol Head Neck Surg. 2017; 3(2):92–96

[20] Ong AA, Murphey AW, Nguyen SA, et al. Efficacy of upper airway stimulation on collapse patterns observed during drug-induced sedation endoscopy. Otolaryngol Head Neck Surg. 2016; 154(5):970–977

[21] Hasselbacher K, Seitz A, Abrams N, Wollenberg B, Steffen A. Complete concentric collapse at the soft palate in sleep endoscopy: what change is possible after UPPP in patients with CPAP failure? Sleep Breath. 2018; 22(4):933–938

21 Pediatric Sleep Endoscopy

An Boudewyns and Palma Benedek

Abstract

Drug induced sedation endoscopy (DISE) is the most commonly used tool to identify the site(s) of upper airway (UA) obstruction in children with obstructive sleep apnea syndrome (OSAS). This technique allows for a dynamic and three-dimensional (3D) evaluation of the entire UA, starting at the nose up to the level of the vocal folds. Although different attempts have been made, there is yet no uniformly accepted protocol for performing DISE in children regarding the drugs used to induce and maintain a state of induced sleep and score the degree and pattern of UA obstruction. Despite these limitations, DISE is now recognized as a meaningful tool in the multidisciplinary management of children with comorbid conditions, contributing to OSAS in children with persistent disease following (adeno)tonsillectomy (AT) and in children with small tonsils. Expanding indications are its use in surgically naive children with OSAS as well as in infants and young children. Future challenges include the development of a universally accepted protocol for pediatric DISE. In addition, outcome measures of DISE directed management, surgical and non-surgical, should be defined and collected.

Keywords: children, infant, upper airway, adenotonsillectomy, obstructive sleep apnea syndrome, endoscopy

21.1 Introduction

Obstructive sleep apnea syndrome (OSAS) is a common condition affecting 1 to 4% of otherwise healthy children,[1] with increasing prevalence rates in subgroups such as children with Down syndrome,[2] obesity,[3] and children with craniofacial malformations, complex abnormalities or neuromuscular conditions.[1] Adenotonsillar hypertrophy is the key feature in many children with OSAS, and adenotonsillectomy (AT) is the first-line treatment in pediatric OSAS. The success rate of AT in otherwise healthy and nonobese children is 75%.[1] Early identification and adequate management of children with residual disease is required to prevent long-term morbidity.[4] Persistent OSAS following AT may be caused by the preoperative existence of risk factors for persistent disease such as severe OSAS at baseline or the presence of comorbidities. During the past years, the possibility of persistent upper airway (UA) obstruction at levels other than the adenotonsillar region has been increasingly recognized as a cause for persistent OSAS in children. Drug-induced sedation endoscopy (DISE) and cine magnetic resonance imaging (MRI) are the most commonly used tools for UA evaluation and identification of sites of persistent UA obstruction in children with persistent disease.[5]

Croft et al can be considered pioneers of pediatric DISE. In 1990, these authors published their experience with flexible nasendoscopy under light anesthesia in 15 children with OSAS.[6] Myatt and Beckenham proposed sleep nasendoscopy combined with rigid laryngobronchoscopy to be included in the standard workup of children with complex UA obstruction such as those with severe OSAS, children with persistent OSAS despite previous AT, and children with OSAS requiring but unable to tolerate continuous positive airway pressure (CPAP).[7] Despite these two promising initial publications, it was only during the last 8 years that pediatric DISE gained interest among clinicians treating children with OSAS. An increasing number of publications on DISE in children pointed toward several unsolved issues such as the lack of a uniform scoring system and anesthetic protocol. There is yet no consensus whether all children with OSAS, only a subgroup should undergo DISE, or whether DISE-directed surgery improves treatment outcomes.[8,9]

The aims of this chapter are to provide an overview of the different UA regions that should be addressed during DISE; describe different scoring systems; and discuss indications for DISE in children and the outcomes of DISE-directed surgery. Finally, some clinical case scenarios will be presented, illustrating the role of DISE in different subgroups of children with OSAS.

21.2 Sites of Potential UA Obstruction in Children

The introduction of a slim, flexible endoscope in the UA allows for a systematic evaluation of all possible sites of UA obstruction, starting at the nostrils and up to the vocal folds (▶ Fig. 21.1).

21.2.1 The Nose and Nasopharynx

The nasal passages should be assessed for turbinate hypertrophy or nasal septal deviation. At the level of the nasopharynx, one should look for adenoid hypertrophy. ▶ Fig. 21.2 commonly used grading systems are based upon how much of the nasopharynx is occupied by the adenoid. DISE assessment of adenoid size is highly correlated with indirect mirror nasopharyngoscopy at the time of surgery and was found to provide a reliable diagnosis of adenoid hypertrophy prior to adenoidectomy.[10] Adenoid regrowth was observed during DISE in 44.6% of

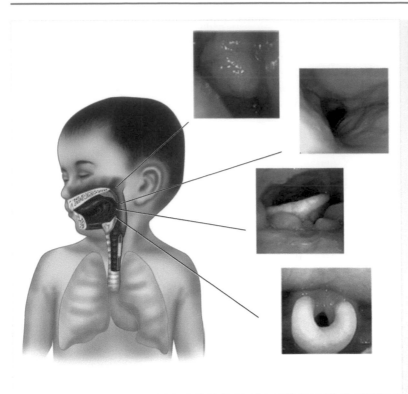

Fig. 21.1 During pediatric DISE, a thin flexible endoscope (pediatric endoscope) is passed through the nostril up to the level of the vocal folds to assess the UA for potential site(s) of UA obstruction or collapse. Abbreviations: UA, upper airway; DISE, drug-induced sleep endoscopy.

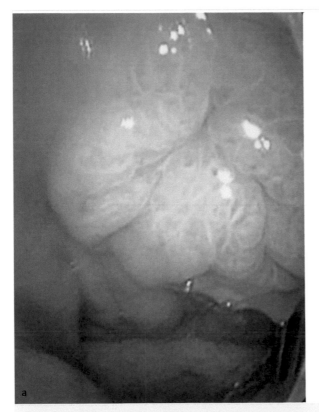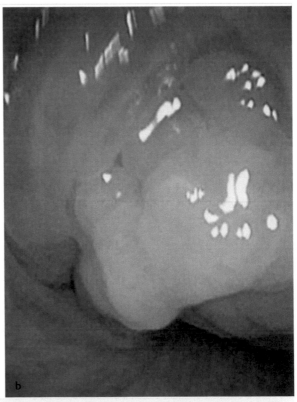

Fig. 21.2 Evaluation of the nasopharynx. Adenoids causing 25% (a) and complete (b) obstruction of the nasopharynx.

children with a mean age of 7.1 years and persistent OSAS documented by polysomnography (PSG).[11]

An anteroposterior (AP) collapse of the palate onto the adenoids or the posterior pharyngeal wall may cause UA obstruction at this level.

21.2.2 Oropharynx: Tonsils and Lateral Pharyngeal Wall

The oropharynx will show dynamic changes, according to the respiratory cycle, with narrowing during inspiration and expansion during expiration. However, in normal circumstances, the passage of airflow should not be obstructed at this level. Narrowing in latero-lateral direction may be caused by tonsillar hypertrophy and/or medialization of the lateral pharyngeal walls, resulting in a central crowding of the oropharynx. Tonsillar obstruction may manifest as tonsils are touching each other at the midline of the oropharynx. In young children with a typically high-positioned larynx, a compression of the epiglottis between the tonsils may be observed (► Fig. 21.3a, b).

In children with small tonsils or tonsils lying deep in the tonsillar fossa, medialization of the lateral pharyngeal walls may result in a similar central crowding of the UA.[1,2] In children without prior tonsillectomy and especially in those with small tonsils on clinical examination, it might prove difficult to separate the relative contribution of the tonsils and lateral pharyngeal walls but complete airway obstruction during DISE may be observed in children with grade 1 tonsils (► Fig. 21.3c).[13]

Among children with neurodevelopmental hypotonia a circumferential narrowing of the oropharynx may be observed caused by a collapse of the pharyngeal tissues.[12]

A significant correlation was found between Brodsky tonsil score and the degree of tonsillar obstruction observed during DISE in a study of children undergoing DISE prior to AT.[14] Similarly, a positive correlation was found between tonsil size and scores for lateral pharyngeal wall collapse, with a linear 0.7 point increase in lateral pharyngeal wall collapse for each 1-point increase in tonsil size.[15]

21.2.3 Tongue Base

Evaluation of the tongue base should include an assessment of lingual tonsillar hypertrophy. Collapse of the tongue base against the posterior pharyngeal wall may be a primary condition or result from mandibular hypoplasia. Mandibular hypoplasia is a typical finding in children with Pierre Robin sequence, oculo–auriculo–vertebral (OAV) spectrum, Treacher Collins syndrome, and other syndromic conditions in which a relatively small mandible does not allow for a correct position of the tongue in the airway, resulting in glossoptosis (► Fig. 21.4).

Lingual tonsillar hypertrophy has been increasingly recognized as a cause of UA obstruction and unanticipated

difficult intubation. Lingual tonsillar hypertrophy will result in crowding of the vallecula by lymphoid tissue. The cause of lingual tonsillar hypertrophy is unknown but chronic infection, gastroesophageal reflux, and compensatory mechanism following earlier AT may play a role.

A maneuver such as a jaw thrust or chin-lift may be helpful to differentiate between lingual tonsillar hypertrophy and glossoptosis (► Fig. 21.5).[16]

21.2.4 Epiglottis

At the level of the epiglottis, it is important to distinguish between a primary collapse of the epiglottis against the pharyngeal wall and a secondary collapse of the epiglottis being pushed posteriorly by the tongue base, as described by Yellon et al.[17] In children with neurodevelopmental hypotonia, a circumferential collapse of the UA at the level of the epiglottis concurrent with a tongue base collapse may be observed (► Fig. 21.6).[12]

21.2.5 Supraglottis– Sleep-Dependent or Late Onset Laryngomalacia

Supraglottic obstruction may be caused by an inspiratory collapse of prominent mucosal folds on the accessory cartilages above the arytenoids. This phenomenon resembles infantile laryngomalacia without curling of the epiglottis and was first described by Richter et al.[18] This form of laryngomalacia typically occurs in older children and is associated with symptoms of OSAS without inspiratory stridor during the day (► Fig. 21.7).

21.2.6 Evaluation of the Lower Airways

Examination of the trachea and bronchi is commonly advocated for children with severe OSAS, especially those with hypotonia because these children are more likely to have multilevel collapse.[8]

The majority of children with moderate to severe OSAS and those with persistent OSAS have multiple sites of UA obstruction.[13,14]

21.3 Drug Used for Pediatric DISE

At present, there is no consensus regarding the ideal drug or combination of drugs to be used for pediatric DISE. A complete overview of the different drugs available is out of the scope of this chapter and excellent reviews are available[19,20,21]

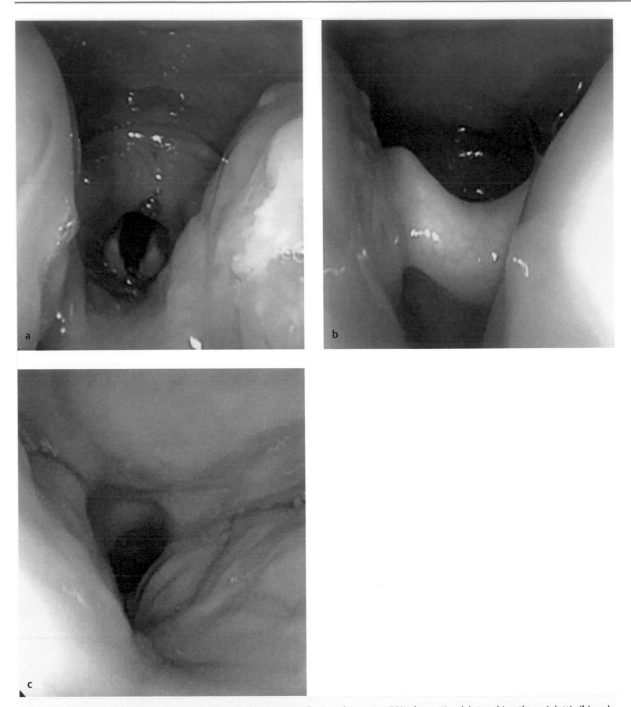

Fig. 21.3 Evaluation of the oropharynx and lateral pharyngeal walls. Tonsils causing 50% obstruction (**a**), touching the epiglottis (**b**) and collapse of the lateral pharyngeal walls in a child with small tonsils on clinical examination (**c**).

The use of topical anesthesia (e.g., lidocaine) is contra-indicated because it may exaggerate findings of laryngo-malacia, reduce UA reflexes, impair the arousal response resulting in increased severity of sleep apnea, and reduce turbinate volume.

Most children require an inhalational anesthetic at the beginning of the procedure in order to insert an IV line. It is recommended that inhalational anesthetics be discontinued as soon as IV access is obtained, because they may decrease UA muscle activity and confound findings during DISE.

Propofol is typically used in adult studies and many reports on pediatric DISE[14,22] but this drug has a dose-dependent effect on the UA by increasing UA collapsibility

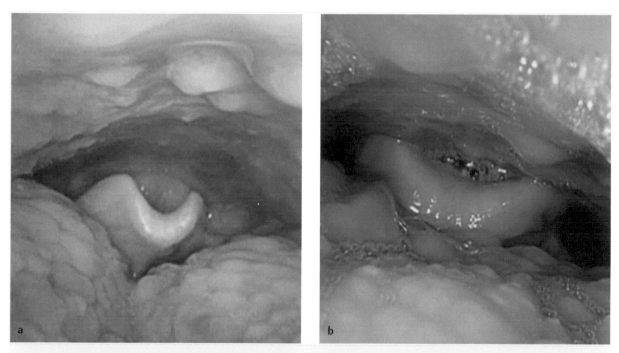

Fig. 21.4 (**a, b**) Evaluation of the tongue base. Normal position of the tongue base and epiglottis, and partial anteroposterior obstruction at the tongue base, causing a collapse of the epiglottis against the posterior pharyngeal wall.

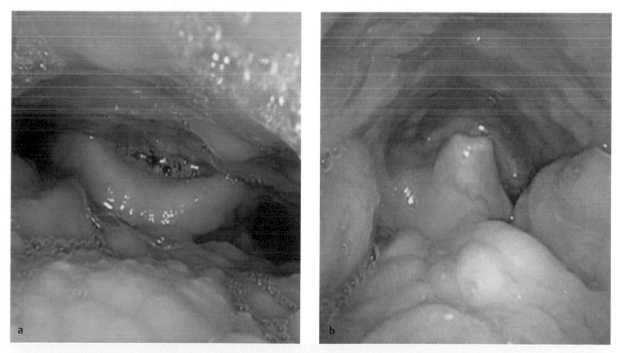

Fig. 21.5 Lingual tonsils. Tongue base obstruction caused by lingual tonsillar hypertrophy, becoming manifest after a jaw thrust maneuver (compare baseline situation in **a** with **b**).

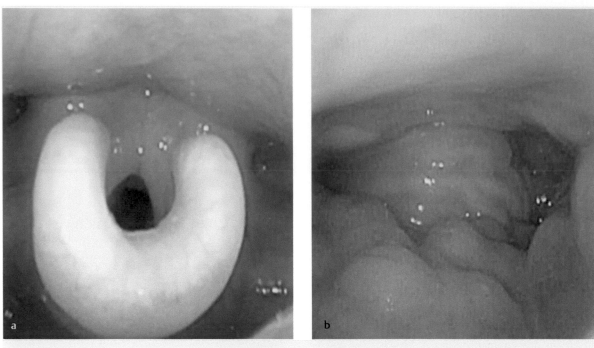

Fig. 21.6 (a, b) Epiglottis. Normal position of the epiglottis and primary collapse of the epiglottis against the posterior pharyngeal wall, with normal position of the tongue base.

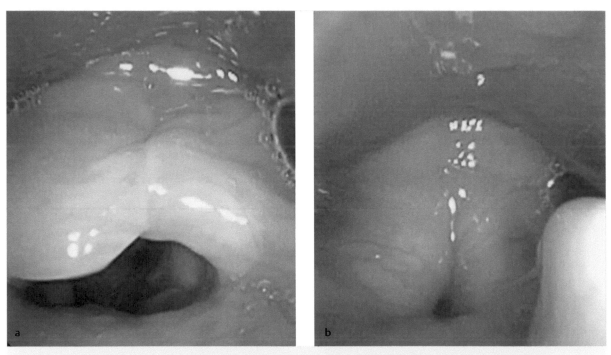

Fig. 21.7 Laryngomalacia. Late onset laryngomalacia with a partial (**a**) and complete (**b**) inspiratory collapse of redundant supra-arythenoidal mucosa.

and decreasing genioglossus muscle tone.[20,21] Infants and toddlers may be at increased risk for UA obstruction and desaturation than older children under propofol sedation.[23] A close titration of propofol to avoid false-positive results exaggerating UA collapse and prevent UA obstruction is thus required.[21] The neuropharmacological profile of dexmedetomidine (DEX) seems very promising, because it promotes a more natural sleep architecture without respiratory depressant effect. A combination of DEX and ketamine is used by many pediatric sleep surgeons, because of a lower risk of respiratory depression and fewer oxygen desaturations below 85% compared to propofol alone or a combination of propofol and sevoflurane.[24] DEX may result in transient changes in blood pressure and heart rate[25,26] and has a longer onset of action and increased drug clearance compared to propofol.[21] DEX is not licensed in Europe for use in children.

21.4 Indications for DISE

Indications for DISE in children are evolving. Commonly accepted indications for DISE in children[9] and expanding indications are summarized in ▶ Table 21.1 and will be discussed in sections 21.4.1 and 21.4.2.

21.4.1 Commonly Accepted Indications for DISE in Children

Persistent OSA after Denotonsillectomy

DISE and cine MRI are the most commonly used tools to identify the site(s) of UA obstruction in children with persistent OSAS following AT.[5] Papers on the use of pediatric DISE for this indication originate from multiple institutions, and DISE is more widely used and accepted as a tool for UA evaluation in children with persistent OSAS.[5,8,9] Most children with persistent OSAS have multiple sites of airway obstruction. Adenoid regrowth

was observed in 44.6% of children with persistent disease when DISE was performed at a mean of 1.75 years following the initial adenoidectomy.[11] However, the authors emphasized that adenoid regrowth is unlikely to be the sole site of persistent airway obstruction and that most of the patients in their series required an additional procedure next to revision adenoidectomy to resolve their airway obstruction. Tongue base obstruction with/without lingual tonsillar hypertrophy and laryngomalacia are the most common causes of persistent disease, especially in children with comorbidities.[5,27] Some authors identified inferior turbinate hypertrophy as a contributor to persistent disease.[16,28]

Prior to AT in Patients at Risk for Persistent Disease

AT is less successful in a large subgroup of children: those with severe OSAS. Some children present comorbid conditions that may contribute to their OSAS such conditions that could affect UA muscle tone or adversely affect neurologic status or anatomic abnormalities associated with UA obstruction. In these children, it has been demonstrated that there is no correlation between tonsil size and apnea–hypopnea index (AHI), indicating that the site of UA obstruction may be at another level.[15] These children are more likely to present multilevel UA obstruction, and DISE may be a useful tool to guide treatment beyond AT.[7] Studies have demonstrated the value of DISE in children with Down syndrome,[29] Prader Willy syndrome,[30] Apert and Crouzon syndromes,[31] and hypotonia.[32]

Significant Symptoms of OSAS or OSAS with Small Tonsils and Adenoids (Disproportion)

The best management of OSAS in children without tonsillar hypertrophy is unknown. Even in a multidisciplinary

Table 21.1 Commonly accepted, and expanding indications for DISE in children

Proposed indications[9]	Expanding indications
Persistent OSAS after adenotonsillectomy	Prior to adenotonsillectomy in otherwise healthy children with OSAS
Prior to adenotonsillectomy in patients at high-risk for persistent OSAS such as obesity, Down syndrome, craniofacial anomalies and neurological impairment	Infants and young children (<2 years old)
Significant symptoms of OSAS or OSAS with small tonsils and adenoids (disproportion)	
Suspicion of sleep-dependent laryngomalacia	
Prior to hypoglossal nerve stimulator treatment	

Abbreviation: OSAS, obstructive sleep apnea syndrome.

UA center involving different pediatric subspecialties, only about one-third of decisions regarding the management of children with OSAS without tonsillar hypertrophy is evidence based.[33]

Miller et al demonstrated that the majority of children with OSAS and a Brodsky score of 1 did not demonstrate lateral pharyngeal wall obstruction and that evaluation for other sites of obstruction may be warranted in these children.[15] Adenoid hypertrophy and tongue base obstruction were identified as the most common sites of obstruction in patients with small tonsils.[15] Children with discordant results between clinical examination and PSG (i.e., children with OSAS and small tonsils or children with severe OSAS regardless of tonsillar size) are considered candidates for DISE, although the definition of "disproportionate" OSAS may vary.

Some authors use the label "disproportional" to describe a group of children with small tonsils (Friedman tonsil score <3) and AHI ≥3/hr without previous OSAS surgery or AHI > 10/hr.[22] Multilevel obstruction requiring additional surgery was found in 30.2% of the patients, with Friedman disproportion supporting a role for DISE in identifying these additional sites of UA obstruction. The authors also suggest that some of the children with persistent OSAS may have been disproportional patients, who were treated as conventional ones by AT, despite having (unidentified) multilevel obstruction.

Small tonsils during DISE were found to be an independent predictor of treatment failure in a series of 207 otherwise healthy patients undergoing DISE-directed surgery for sleep-disordered breathing (SDB) (AT, tonsillectomy or adenoidectomy). The data should be interpreted with some caution because OSAS outcome was based on parental resolution of symptoms evaluated by the modified pediatric sleep questionnaire (PSQ).[34]

Suspicion of Sleep-Dependent Laryngomalacia

Sleep-dependent laryngomalacia was first described by Richter et al.[18] This condition was typically seen in school-aged children and presents as obstruction at the arytenoids and supra-arytenoid mucosa with a normal appearing epiglottis and normal ary-epiglottic folds. Clinical improvement is seen after supraglottoplasty, with trimming of the supra-arytenoid tissue. These children typically do not present with stridor but with OSAS-related symptoms. Prevalence rates of 3.9 to 5.4% have been reported in children without prior history of AT[14,35] and it represents a common cause of persistent OSAS.[5]

Prior to Hypoglossal Nerve Stimulator Treatment

Studies in adults have shown that patient with complete AP or lateral soft palate collapse and/or collapse of the epiglottis are at increased risk of treatment failure following UA stimulation.[36] DISE was used in the first paper on UA stimulation in children to confirm that none of the included patients presented with circumferential collapse at the velum, since this is considered a contraindication for UA stimulation.[37]

21.4.2 Expanding Indications for Pediatric DISE

As the clinical experience with pediatric DISE is growing, new indications are emerging.

Prior to AT in Otherwise Healthy Children with OSAS

AT is the first-line treatment for pediatric OSAS with a success rate of 71 to 87% in a normally developing pediatric population.[38,39] These observations prompted researchers to investigate whether DISE performed before AT in these children would affect treatment decision-making. Although some studies are in favor of DISE prior to AT, this is still not uniformly accepted.[8,40,41] Gazzaz et al performed a study including 550 patients aged 3 to 17 years without prior surgery[42]. Surgical decision-making was affected by findings during DISE in 35% of the patients. Despite the high number of included patients in this study, a disadvantage is the lack of PSG to confirm the diagnosis of OSAS, which was based upon pulse oximetry and modified PSQ.

Boudewyns et al performed DISE in a group of 37 otherwise healthy children, age 4.1 (2.1–6.0) years with moderate-to-severe OSAS and AHI 9.0/hr (6.1–19.3), which was documented by PSG.[14] In this study, nonsurgical treatment was proposed in 11% of the children, based upon UA findings during DISE. A more recent paper from the same group found that DISE prior to AT in otherwise healthy patients altered the therapeutic decision-making in ⅓rd of infants and ¼th of children with OSAS.[43] It should be noted, however, that the infants and children included in this paper had severe OSAS and all the children receiving non-AT treatment had multilevel collapse. Collu et al found that DISE changed the management in a "conventional OSAS" group in only 4.5% of the cases. Notably, conventional OSAS was defined as no previous surgery for OSAS and AHI ≤ 10/hr with variable Friedman tonsil size. Further studies investigating the role of DISE in surgically naive children with OSAS should take OSAS severity and comorbidity into account. Children with more severe OSAS and those with comorbidity are more likely to have multiple sites of UA obstruction, and DISE in these patients may be helpful to guide personalized treatment and limit comorbidity from unnecessary or surgery deemed to be unsuccessful.

DISE in Infants and Young Children (< 2 years of Age)

Young infants and children have a high-incidence of multilevel and dynamic UA collapse including pharyngeal wall collapse, and collapse of the epiglottis and laryngomalacia.[44] In addition, infants and young children with OSAS more often have an underlying condition, predisposing to UA obstruction.[45] Croft and colleagues were the first to describe the value of endoscopic evaluation and treatment of sleep-associated UA obstruction in infants and young children.[6] Already in 1990, these authors emphasized the importance of thorough UA evaluation when considering surgery in infants and young children with OSAS.[6]

Although few data are available in literature, DISE seems a promising tool for UA evaluation and treatment selection in these young patients with OSAS.[45,46]

21.5 DISE Protocol

DISE in children is typically performed with the child in the operating theatre. The child is positioned supine with the head in a neutral position (no pillows or head rest) and full cardiorespiratory monitoring is carried out in attendance of a pediatric anesthesiologist. A flexible fiberoptic endoscope is introduced via the nose into the UA to assess the different levels as described above. Some clinicians include a chin-lift or jaw-thrust maneuver during the procedure to assess closed-mouth breathing (chin-lift) or the effect of mandibular repositioning (jawthrust).[9] Some authors advocate the use of BIS (bispectral Index) monitoring to measure the depth of anesthesia and the ideal moment to assess the UA. BIS levels between 60 and 70 may be the most informative.[16]

When UA surgery is performed immediately after DISE, parental consent for different surgical interventions should be obtained prior to the examination. Some clinicians have criticized this approach as it would make operative planning more difficult and reduce the input of families in a shared decision-making process. Advantages include the increased convenience and reduced anesthesia exposure when airway evaluation can be combined with a surgical intervention, targeting the site of UA obstruction. In daily practice, we believe that straightforward surgical procedures such as turbinate reduction and AT could be performed during the same anesthesia. More complex interventions on the other hand like tongue base surgery or supraglottoplasty are preferentially performed at a second stage, since these require more extensive counseling and a different postoperative management.

21.6 DISE Scoring Systems

The velum, oropharynx, tongue base and epiglottis (VOTE) classification is the most popular scoring system especially for adults[47] and also widely used for children.[9] The VOTE classification analyses the severity and configuration of obstruction at four anatomical levels: velum, oropharynx, tongue base and epiglottis.[48] In children, information regarding obstruction at the nasopharynx, including the adenoids and supraglottis, is also required. Some scoring systems also add information on turbinate hypertrophy. Different scoring systems have been used for DISE in children but none of them is universally accepted.[9] Boudewyns et al published a scoring system including six different UA sites and divided them into fixed obstruction (adenoids, tonsils, tongue base) and dynamic collapse at the level of palate, epiglottis, laryngomalacia, and circumferential narrowing at the level of the oropharynx or hypopharynx (labeled as hypotonia). Fixed obstructions are scored quantitatively according to the severity of obstruction, whereas dynamic collapse is scored as present or absent.

This scoring system is illustrated in ▶ Table 21.2. The Chan–Parikh classification system allows to calculate a total obstructive score, which was found to correlate with OSAS severity (preprocedural AHI and oxygen nadir).[49,50]

The ideal system should include all possible sites of UA obstruction, be simple and practical, and have a high inter- and intrarater reliability. In addition, it should quantify not only the presence but also the severity of the UA obstruction at different UA levels.

21.7 Outcome of DISE-Directed Surgery in Children

An important clinical question is whether DISE-directed surgery in children improves clinical outcome. This has been studied in different pediatric populations.

21.7.1 Surgically Naive, Healthy Patients with OSAS

Boudewyns et al reported on a group of infants and children with severe OSAS documented by PSG, without significant comorbidity and no prior surgery for OSAS.[43] Patients were divided into two groups according to the type of DISE-directed surgery: those undergoing AT and those undergoing another treatment than AT (e.g., adenoidectomy, tonsillectomy, CPAP). Outcomes in terms of successful treatment (posttreatment obstructive AHI < 5/hr) and cure (posttreatment AHI < 2/hr) were not significantly different in both groups. The authors concluded that DISE may allow for individually tailored treatment, avoiding unnecessary surgery, with similar outcomes to standard treatment by AT.

Alsufyani et al investigated clinical and DISE variables that may predict failure of DISE-directed adenoidectomy and/or tonsillectomy in 382 otherwise healthy children with OSAS.[34] Diagnosis of OSAS was based upon clinical findings, modified PSQ and pulse oximetry, and treat-

Table 21.2 Scoring sheet for pediatric DISE[14]

Scoring sheet pediatric DISE			
Name: ...;		Diagnosis: ...	
First name: ...;		Previous surgery: ...	
Birth date: ...;		Comorbidity: ...	
Examination date: ...;		Examinator: ...	
Anesthesia: sevoflurane + propofol/propofol only			
Propofol dosage: ...mg/kg/hr			

Fixed obstruction		Dynamic collapse	
Level	Findings	Level	Findings
Adenoids	0 = (none) 1 = <50% obstruction 2 = 50% up to 75% obstruction 3 = >75% obstruction	Palate	0 = no collapse 1 = collapse present
Tonsils	0 = none 1 = <50% obstruction 2 = 50 to 90% obstruction 3 = tonsils touch at midline	Epiglottis*	0 = no collapse 1 = collapse present
Tongue base	0 = none 1 = partial obstruction 2 = complete obstruction	Hypotonia	0 = absent 1 = present
		Laryngomalacia	0 = absent 1 = present
Additional comments/findings:			

* Epiglottis pulled backward by the tonsils or tongue base is not considered as dynamic epiglottis collapse.

ment failure was based on parental report (PSQ > 33%). Thirty-two percent of the patients had persistent disease and 89% of the patients who failed treatment had an alternative diagnosis on DISE apart from adenotonsillar hypertrophy. Findings during DISE of chronic rhinitis, deviated nasal septum, and tonsil size (small tonsils) were independent predictors of treatment failure.

21.7.2 Children with Persistent OSAS with/without Comorbidity

Children with comorbidity are more likely to present persistent OSAS following AT, and most studies on DISE-directed surgery in children with persistent OSAS included children with comorbidities.

In one of the first papers on pediatric DISE in children by Myatt et al, eight out of 20 patients had prepostoperative PSG.[7] Five had associated comorbidity (cerebral palsy, Down syndrome, Pierre Robin sequence). These authors observed a significant improvement in AHI from a mean

of 48 ± 15.5/hr to 4.6 ± 4.5/hr. In addition, it was observed that the site of UA obstruction may vary among children with the same syndrome, explaining why some treatments may succeed in some children and fail in others.

Wootten et al presented subjective and objective outcomes on DISE-directed surgery in a group of 26 consecutive children who failed AT.[27] About half of them (51%) had trisomy 21. The subjects underwent a variety of DISE-directed procedures, resulting in a subjective improvement in 92%. Eleven patients had a prepostop PSG, showing a significant improvement in AHI.

He et al reported the outcomes of DISE-directed surgery in a heterogeneous group of 56 patients (55 with comorbidity), comprising 21 infants and 35 children without tonsillar hypertrophy (previous AT).[51] A large variety of procedures was performed and 39% were treated with > 1 procedure selected by the surgeon based upon DISE findings. The infants were significantly less likely to undergo adenoidectomy or lingual tonsillectomy but more commonly treated by supraglottoplasty.

A significant improvement in postoperative AHI was found in the infants and not in the children with OSAS without tonsillar hypertrophy; however, both groups improved in saturation nadir. Nevertheless, the likelihood of a posttreatment AHI < 5/hr was not affected by history of previous tonsillectomy, age or performance of supraglottoplasty, and DISE-directed surgery was more effective in children with lower AHI. Overall, 44% of the included patients had a postoperative AHI < 5/hr following DISE-directed surgery.

21.7.3 Children with Hypotonia

Dynamic UA abnormalities are very common in hypotonic children independent of age.[44] Park et al investigated the outcomes of DISE-directed surgery in 87 children with syndromic or nonsyndromic hypotonia and neuromuscular dysfunction and found that 31% had trisomy 21.[32] DISE revealed multilevel obstruction in 49% and among children with previous AT, all had significant obstruction at the tongue base, and 73% had significant obstruction at the supraglottis. Most children underwent one procedure and the most common procedures were AT (80%), supraglottoplasty (18%) and lingual tonsillectomy (11.5%). Prepostoperative PSG was available for 26 children and showed a significant improvement in AHI and oxygen nadir along with a significant improvement in quality of life. However, residual OSAS is common in this population, with an average postoperative AHI of 11.8/hr.

21.7.4 Children with Down Syndrome

Children with Down syndrome are often included in studies on the role of DISE in children with persistent disease or hypotonia. Maris et al reported DISE findings and outcome of DISE-directed surgery in a cohort of 41 young, nonobese and surgically naive children with Down syndrome.[29] Multilevel UA collapse was found in 85.4% with a high-prevalence of epiglottic collapse (49%) and laryngomalacia (12%). Only about 25% had tongue base obstruction, a finding that is likely different in children with Down syndrome and previous UA surgery. DISE-directed surgery was performed in 25 and consisted of AT, tonsillectomy or adenoidectomy. Five out of these 25 surgically treated patients had a multilevel collapse and treatment resulted in a significant improvement in AHI and mean oxygen saturation. Despite these improvements, residual OSAS with an AHI ≥ 5/hr was present in 52%.

21.8 Clinical Case Scenarios

21.8.1 Case 1

A 7-year-old boy was admitted to the sleep clinic because of parental concern regarding snoring, witnessed apneas, and struggling to breathe during sleep. He did not experience any difficulties to fall asleep, but occasionally woke up during the night. His symptoms persisted despite an AT performed one year earlier. According to the parental report, his snoring had intensified, and the number and duration of the apneas worsened during the last 6 months.

He did not have any other sleep problems such as sleeping terrors, nightmares, leg movements, sleep paralysis, or cataplexy. He showed no daytime symptoms (e.g., attention deficit, hyperactivity). The boy usually enjoyed school, and practiced sports on a daily basis. Clinical examination showed inferior turbinate hypertrophy and a Mallampati score III with a high-arched palate. There was no allergy for common respiratory allergens, and body mass index (BMI) percentile was 30%.

Full night PSG showed moderate OSAS with an AHI of 8/hr, desaturation index (DI): 12/hr, and O_2 nadir 75% during REM sleep. DISE was performed because of persistent OSAS (clinical symptoms and abnormal polysomnographic results) in a child with a history of AT. The results of this examination are summarized in ▶ Table 21.3.

In the nasal cavity, the septum was in the midline, and the inferior turbinate was markedly enlarged, touching the septum and blocking the inferior meatus (▶ Fig. 21.8). At the level of the nasopharynx, there was no adenoid regrowth, no obstruction at the level of the tonsils because of earlier tonsillectomy, and no medialization of the lateral pharyngeal walls. DISE showed a partial AP collapse of the tongue base, pushing the epiglottis against the posterior pharyngeal wall (▶ Fig. 21.9). With the jaw-thrust maneuver, the entire region of the true vocal folds could be visualized (▶ Fig. 21.10). There was no laryngomalacia and vocal fold mobility was normal.

Based on these findings, we performed radiofrequency inferior turbinate reduction and the child was referred to an orthodontist with experience in treating pediatric OSAS. Treatment was recommended with rapid maxillary expansion therapy to expand the high-arched palate and the obstruction at the level of the tongue base. Repeat PSG after a 6-month treatment period with rapid maxillary expansion showed a complete resolution of OSAS with an AHI 1/hr, ODI 8/hr and O_2 nadir of 92%.

21.8.2 Case 2

A 4-year-old, obese boy (BMI percentile > 95%) was referred to the sleep clinic because of parental concerns regarding loud snoring, breathing stops and wheezing, especially during periods of UA infection. He was a restless sleeper and the parents mentioned heavy night sweats. He refused going to bed at bedtime, and usually woke up in the middle of the night with a panic attack, screaming and sweating. According to the parental report, he had difficulty getting up in the morning. His afternoon napping time had become longer than earlier. He usually caught UA infections twice a month and had difficulty breathing through his nose. The parents had consulted an ENT surgeon who performed an

Table 21.3 DISE scoring sheet for Case 1

Scoring sheet pediatric DISE				
Name: Patient 1		**Diagnosis:** Moderate OSAS		
Previous surgery: ATE		**Comorbidity:** None		
Anesthesia: Sevoflurane + propofol		**Examinator:** BP		
Propofol dosage: 6 mg/kg/hr				
Fixed obstruction		Dynamic collapse		
Level	Findings	Level	Findings	
Adenoids	0	Palate	0	
Tonsils	0	Epiglottis*	0	
Tongue base	1	Hypotonia	0	
		Laryngomalacia	0	
Additional comments/findings: Markedly enlarged inferior turbinates.				

Abbreviations: DISE, drug-induced sleep endoscopy; OSAS, obstructive sleep apnea syndrome.
* Epiglottis pulled backward by the tonsils or tongue base is not considered as dynamic epiglottis collapse.

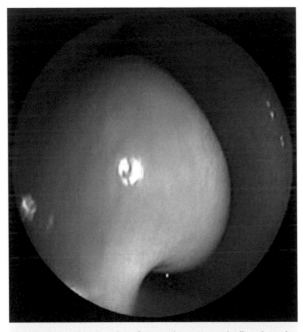

Fig. 21.8 Nasal cavity. The inferior turbinate is markedly enlarged.

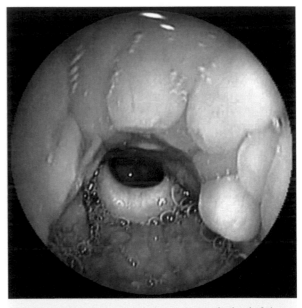

Fig. 21.9 Tongue base. Partial obstruction at the level of the tongue base with secondary collapse of the epiglottis against the posterior pharyngeal wall.

adenoidectomy. In the recovery room, he suffered from severe respiratory distress with severe desaturations, and long periods of apnea ending in a respiratory arrest, which needed reintubation. He recovered in 2 weeks.

Clinical examination revealed hypertrophic tonsils (Brodsky 4+) and obesity. Full night PSG showed severe OSAS with the following values: AHI: 57, 5/hr, ODI: 63/hr,

and O_2 nadir of 57% during REM sleep. CPAP treatment was considered but, before initiation, DISE was performed to investigate whether the child could benefit from additional surgical procedures and the results are presented in ► Table 21.4.

In the nasal cavity, the septum was in the midline and the inferior turbinates were mildly enlarged. There was no obstruction at the level of the adenoids. The tonsils were touching each other and resulting in complete UA obstruction at the level of oropharynx, and the epiglottis was compressed between both tonsils. The level of the tongue base was free in its entirety; both of the true vocal folds were visible by the endoscope positioned at the level of the soft palate. At the level of larynx, late onset laryngomalacia with inspiratory collapse of redundant supra-arytenoidal mucosa

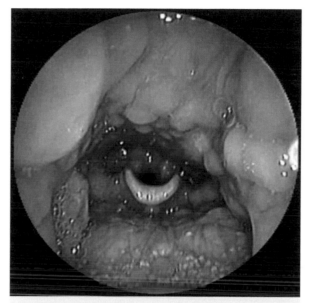

Fig. 21.10 Jaw thrust maneuver. During jaw thrust, the entire region of the true vocal folds is visualized.

was present (▶ Fig. 21.11). Vocal fold mobility was normal. Taking into account the age of the child, the results of polysomnography, DISE findings and counseling of the parents, a tonsillectomy was performed. The child was transferred to the pediatric intensive care unit (PICU) during the postoperative period.

During the first postoperative 24 hours, desaturations occurred but these resolved spontaneously. The next day, he was discharged from the PICU to the ENT department. After a month, the patient's symptoms resolved and the PSG test showed AHI: 1/hr. These findings suggest a resolution of late onset laryngomalacia following tonsillectomy as reported in earlier studies.[35,43] Although the exact mechanism is unknown, the observed improvement may result from a decrease in negative pressure at the laryngeal level, following relief of obstruction more upstream in the UA.

21.9 Role of DISE in the Multidisciplinary and Integrated Approach to Pediatric OSAS

Obstruction of the UA during sleep is one of the key features of pediatric OSAS, and DISE is a valuable tool for identifying the site(s) of UA obstruction. Therefore, its role as a selection tool for UA surgery has been investigated. Whether DISE also may play a role in the selection of nonsurgical treatment such as orthodontic treatment or CPAP and noninvasive ventilation has received little attention until now. However, similarly to data reported in adults, it

Table 21.4 DISE scoring sheet for Case 2

Scoring sheet pediatric DISE					
Name: Patient 2			**Diagnosis:** Severe OSAS		
Previous surgery: Adenoidectomy			**Comorbidity:** Obesity		
Anesthesia: Sevoflurane + propofol			**Examinator:** BP		
Propofol dosage: 6 mg/kg/hr					
Fixed obstruction			Dynamic collapse		
Level	Findings		Level	Findings	
Adenoids	0		Palate	0	
Tonsils	3		Epiglottis*	1	
Tongue base	0		Hypotonia	1	
			Laryngomalacia	1	

Additional comments/finding: Inferior turbinates mildly enlarged.

Abbreviations: DISE, drug-induced sleep endoscopy; OSAS, obstructive sleep apnea syndrome.
* Epiglottis pulled backward by the tonsils or tongue base is not considered as dynamic epiglottis collapse.

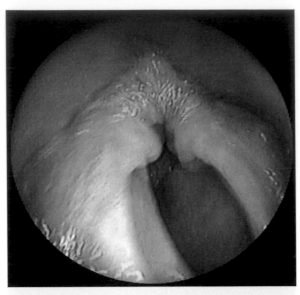

Fig. 21.11 Lateonset laryngomalacia. Late onset laryngomalacia with inspiratory collapse of redundant supra-arytenoid mucosa.

is conceivable that DISE could also be used to guide nonsurgical treatment. Therefore, it may become an important tool in the hands of the ENT surgeon for personalized treatment, either surgical or nonsurgical, in an individual child. However, the management of pediatric OSAS, especially in children with persistent disease, associated comorbidity, infants and young children, should not be based solely on findings during DISE. A stepwise approach to the diagnosis and management of OSAS in children, infants and young children has been proposed, taking into account several other factors such as the presence of risk factors for OSAS and persistent disease, associated comorbidity resulting from OSAS, and underlying conditions contributing to OSAS and OSAS severity.[1,45] In addition, patient and parental preferences, treatment compliance and experience of the treating surgeon with different UA procedures should be considered. It is now recognized that the management of pediatric OSAS relies on a multidisciplinary approach, requiring an input from different pediatric subspecialties and taking into account the available scientific evidence. This concept is summarized in ▸ Fig. 21.12.

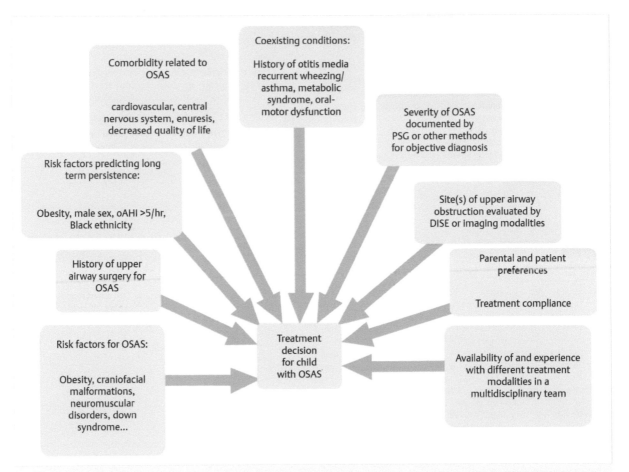

Fig. 21.12 Integrated and personalized approach for the treatment of OSAS in children. Abbreviation: OSAS, obstructive sleep apnea syndrome.

References

[1] Kaditis AG, Alonso Alvarez ML, Boudewyns A, et al. Obstructive sleep disordered breathing in 2- to 18-year-old children: diagnosis and management. Eur Respir J. 2016; 47(1):69–94

[2] Maris M, Verhulst S, Wojciechowski M, Van de Heyning P, Boudewyns A. Prevalence of obstructive sleep apnea in children with down syndrome. Sleep (Basel). 2016; 39(3):699–704

[3] Verhulst SL, Schrauwen N, Haentjens D, et al. Sleep-disordered breathing in overweight and obese children and adolescents: prevalence, characteristics and the role of fat distribution. Arch Dis Child. 2007; 92(3):205–208

[4] Boudewyns A, Abel F, Alexopoulos E, et al. Adenotonsillectomy to treat obstructive sleep apnea: is it enough? Pediatr Pulmonol. 2017; 52(5):699–709

[5] Manickam PV, Shott SR, Boss EF, et al. Systematic review of site of obstruction identification and non-CPAP treatment options for children with persistent pediatric obstructive sleep apnea. Laryngoscope. 2016; 126(2):491–500

[6] Croft CB, Thomson HG, Samuels MP, Southall DP. Endoscopic evaluation and treatment of sleep-associated upper airway obstruction in infants and young children. Clin Otolaryngol Allied Sci. 1990; 15(3): 209–216

[7] Myatt HM, Beckenham EJ. The use of diagnostic sleep nasendoscopy in the management of children with complex upper airway obstruction. Clin Otolaryngol Allied Sci. 2000; 25(3):200–208

[8] Friedman NR, Parikh SR, Ishman SL, et al. The current state of pediatric drug-induced sleep endoscopy. Laryngoscope. 2017; 127 (1):266–272

[9] Wilcox LJ, Bergeron M, Reghunathan S, Ishman SL. An updated review of pediatric drug-induced sleep endoscopy. Laryngoscope Investig Otolaryngol. 2017; 2(6):423–431

[10] Zalzal HG, Carr M, Kohler W, Coutras SW. Adenoid size by drug induced sleep endoscopy compared to nasopharyngeal mirror exam. Int J Pediatr Otorhinolaryngol. 2018; 112:75–79

[11] Zalzal HG, Carr M, Nanda N, Coutras S. Drug induced sleep endoscopy identification of adenoid regrowth in pediatric obstructive sleep apnea. Int J Otolaryngol. 2018; 2018.7920907

[12] Truong MT, Woo VG, Koltai PJ. Sleep endoscopy as a diagnostic tool in pediatric obstructive sleep apnea. Int J Pediatr Otorhinolaryngol. 2012; 76(5):722–727

[13] Ulualp SO, Szmuk P. Drug-induced sleep endoscopy for upper airway evaluation in children with obstructive sleep apnea. Laryngoscope. 2013; 123(1):292–297

[14] Boudewyns A, Verhulst S, Maris M, Saldien V, Van de Heyning P. Drug-induced sedation endoscopy in pediatric obstructive sleep apnea syndrome. Sleep Med. 2014; 15(12):1526–1531

[15] Miller C, Purcell PL, Dahl JP, et al. Clinically small tonsils are typically not obstructive in children during drug-induced sleep endoscopy. Laryngoscope. 2017; 127(8):1943–1949

[16] Esteller E, Mulas D, Haspert R, Matiñó E, López R, Girabent-Farrés M. Drug-induced sleep-endoscopy in children's sleep related breathing disorders. Acta Otorrinolaringol Esp. 2016; 67(4):212–219

[17] Yellon RF. Epiglottic and base-of-tongue prolapse in children: grading and management. Laryngoscope. 2006; 116(2):194–200

[18] Richter GT, Rutter MJ, deAlarcon A, Orvidas LJ, Thompson DM. Late-onset laryngomalacia: a variant of disease. Arch Otolaryngol Head Neck Surg. 2008; 134(1):75–80

[19] Chatterjee D, Friedman N, Shott S, Mahmoud M. Anesthetic dilemmas for dynamic evaluation of the pediatric upper airway. Semin Cardiothorac Vasc Anesth. 2014; 18(4):371–378

[20] Ehsan Z, Mahmoud M, Shott SR, Amin RS, Ishman SL. The effects of anesthesia and opioids on the upper airway: A systematic review. Laryngoscope. 2016; 126(1):270–284

[21] Shteamer JW, Dedhia RC. Sedative choice in drug-induced sleep endoscopy: A neuropharmacology-based review. Laryngoscope. 2017; 127(1):273–279

[22] Collu MA, Esteller E, Lipari F, et al. A case-control study of Drug-Induced Sleep Endoscopy (DISE) in pediatric population: a proposal for indications. Int J Pediatr Otorhinolaryngol. 2018; 108:113–119

[23] Barbi E, Petaros P, Badina L, et al. Deep sedation with propofol for upper gastrointestinal endoscopy in children, administered by specially trained pediatricians: a prospective case series with emphasis on side effects. Endoscopy. 2006; 38(4):368–375

[24] Kandil A, Subramanyam R, Hossain MM, et al. Comparison of the combination of dexmedetomidine and ketamine to propofol or propofol/sevoflurane for drug-induced sleep endoscopy in children. Paediatr Anaesth. 2016; 26(7):742–751

[25] Jooste EH, Muhly WT, Ibinson JW, et al. Acute hemodynamic changes after rapid intravenous bolus dosing of dexmedetomidine in pediatric heart transplant patients undergoing routine cardiac catheterization. Anesth Analg. 2010; 111(6):1490–1496

[26] Mason KP, Zgleszewski SE, Prescilla R, Fontaine PJ, Zurakowski D. Hemodynamic effects of dexmedetomidine sedation for CT imaging studies. Paediatr Anaesth. 2008; 18(5):393–402

[27] Wootten CT, Chinnadurai S, Goudy SL. Beyond adenotonsillectomy: outcomes of sleep endoscopy-directed treatments in pediatric obstructive sleep apnea. Int J Pediatr Otorhinolaryngol. 2014; 78(7): 1158–1162

[28] Durr ML, Meyer AK, Kezirian EJ, Rosbe KW. Drug-induced sleep endoscopy in persistent pediatric sleep-disordered breathing after adenotonsillectomy. Arch Otolaryngol Head Neck Surg. 2012; 138(7): 638–643

[29] Maris M, Verhulst S, Saldien V, Van de Heyning P, Wojciechowski M, Boudewyns A. Drug-induced sedation endoscopy in surgically naive children with Down syndrome and obstructive sleep apnea. Sleep Med. 2016; 24:63–70

[30] Lan MCHY, Hsu YB, Lan MY, et al. Drug-induced sleep endoscopy in children with Prader-Willi syndrome. Sleep Breath. 2016; 20(3): 1029–1034

[31] Doerga PN, Spruijt B, Mathijssen IM, Wolvius EB, Joosten KF, van der Schroeff MP. Upper airway endoscopy to optimize obstructive sleep apnea treatment in Apert and Crouzon syndromes. J Craniomaxillofac Surg. 2016; 44(2):191–196

[32] Park JS, Chan DK, Parikh SR, Meyer AK, Rosbe KW. Surgical outcomes and sleep endoscopy for children with sleep disordered breathing and hypotonia. Int J Pediatr Otorhinolaryngol. 2016; 90: 99–106

[33] Ishman SL, Tang A, Cohen AP, et al. Decision-making for children with obstructive sleep apnea without tonsillar hypertrophy. Otolaryngol Head Neck Surg. 2016; 154(3):527–531

[34] Alsufyani N, Isaac A, Witmans M, Major P, El-Hakim H. Predictors of failure of DISE-directed adenotonsillectomy in children with sleep disordered breathing. J Otolaryngol Head Neck Surg. 2017; 46(1):37

[35] Thevasagayam M, Rodger K, Cave D, Witmans M, El-Hakim H. Prevalence of laryngomalacia in children presenting with sleep-disordered breathing. Laryngoscope. 2010; 120(8):1662–1666

[36] Ong AA, Murphey AW, Nguyen SA, et al. Efficacy of upper airway stimulation on collapse patterns observed during drug-induced sedation endoscopy. Otolaryngol Head Neck Surg. 2016; 154(5):970–977

[37] Diercks GR, Wentland C, Keamy D, et al. Hypoglossal nerve stimulation in adolescents with down syndrome and obstructive sleep apnea. JAMA Otolaryngol Head Neck Surg. 2017; 144(1):37–42

[38] Ye J, Liu H, Zhang GH, et al. Outcome of adenotonsillectomy for obstructive sleep apnea syndrome in children. Ann Otol Rhinol Laryngol. 2010; 119(8):506–513

[39] Mitchell RB. Adenotonsillectomy for obstructive sleep apnea in children: outcome evaluated by pre- and postoperative polysomnography. Laryngoscope. 2007; 117(10):1844–1854

[40] Galluzzi F, Pignataro L, Gaini RM, Garavello W. Drug induced sleep endoscopy in the decision-making process of children with obstructive sleep apnea. Sleep Med. 2015; 16(3):331–335

[41] Boudewyns A, Verhulst S. Potential role for drug-induced sleep endoscopy (DISE) in paediatric OSA. Sleep Med. 2015; 16(9):1178

[42] Gazzaz MJ, Isaac A, Anderson S, Alsufyani N, Alrajhi Y, El-Hakim H. Does drug-induced sleep endoscopy change the surgical decision in surgically naïve non-syndromic children with snoring/sleep disordered breathing from the standard adenotonsillectomy? A retrospective cohort study. J Otolaryngol Head Neck Surg. 2017; 46(1):12

[43] Boudewyns A, Saldien V, Van de Heyning P, Verhulst S. Drug-induced sedation endoscopy in surgically naïve infants and children with obstructive sleep apnea: impact on treatment decision and outcome. Sleep Breath. 2018; 22(2):503–510

[44] Goldberg S, Shatz A, Picard E, et al. Endoscopic findings in children with obstructive sleep apnea: effects of age and hypotonia. Pediatr Pulmonol. 2005; 40(3):205–210

[45] Kaditis AG, Alonso Alvarez ML, Boudewyns A, et al. ERS statement on obstructive sleep disordered breathing in 1- to 23-month-old children. Eur Respir J. 2017; 50(6):50

[46] Boudewyns A, Van de Heyning P, Verhulst S. Drug-induced sedation endoscopy in children < 2 years with obstructive sleep apnea syndrome: upper airway findings and treatment outcomes. Eur Arch Otorhinolaryngol. 2017; 274(5):2319–2325

[47] Dijemeni E, D'Amone G, Gbati I. Drug-induced sedation endoscopy (DISE) classification systems: a systematic review and meta-analysis. Sleep Breath. 2017; 21(4):983–994

[48] Kezirian EJ, Hohenhorst W, de Vries N. Drug-induced sleep endoscopy: the VOTE classification. Eur Arch Otorhinolaryngol. 2011; 268 (8):1233–1236

[49] Chan DK, Liming BJ, Horn DL, Parikh SR. A new scoring system for upper airway pediatric sleep endoscopy. JAMA Otolaryngol Head Neck Surg. 2014; 140(7):595–602

[50] Dahl JP, Miller C, Purcell PL, et al. Airway obstruction during drug-induced sleep endoscopy correlates with apnea–hypopnea index and oxygen nadir in children. Otolaryngol Head Neck Surg. 2016; 155(4): 676–680

[51] He S, Peddireddy NS, Smith DF, et al. Outcomes of drug-induced sleep endoscopy-directed surgery for pediatric obstructive sleep apnea. Otolaryngol Head Neck Surg. 2018; 158(3):559–565

22 DISE in Children with Craniofacial Anomalies

Paolo G. Morselli, Rossella Sgarzani, Valentina Pinto, Andrea Marzetti, Francesco M. Passali, Nadia Mansouri, P. Vijaya Krishnan, Vikas Agrawal, Srinivas Kishore S, and Ottavio Piccin

Abstract

This chapter focuses on the role of drug-induced sleep endoscopy (DISE) in children with craniofacial anomalies (CFAs). This subgroup of patients may be at increased risk of obstructive sleep apnea (OSA) due to abnormalities in both their facial structure as well as likely upper airway (UA) neuromotor deficits. Although facial skeletal dysmorphology plays a significant role in the etiology of OSA, recent studies have revealed that the obstruction may occur anywhere along the UA. Maxillofacial interventions can be effective in resolving airway obstruction, but in some cases, it is not as successful as is generally thought. Although few data are available in literature, DISE seems to be a promising tool for UA evaluation and treatment selection in this subgroup of children. DISE before surgical treatment may be recommended to identify the exact levels of obstruction and incorporate the findings in the treatment plan, providing a way to tailor better management of OSA in children with CFAs.

Keywords: craniofacial anomalies, sleep-disordered breathing, obstructive sleep apnea, drug-induced sleep endoscopy

22.1 Introduction

Pediatric obstructive sleep apnea (OSA) represents a broad spectrum of diseases resulting from neuromotor dysfunction, lymphoid tissue hypertrophy, and craniofacial skeletal anomalies (CFAs).

In the general pediatric population, it is well known that the frequency of OSA is up to 4% with a peak between 2 to 6 years of age when adenotonsillar size is largest relative to airway size.[1]

Craniofacial skeletal morphology plays an important role in the patency of the upperairway (UA) in both healthy children and children with CFAs, and consequently children with craniofacial conditions are generally at increased risk for development of OSA.[2]

The reported prevalence of OSA in children with craniofacial syndromes ranges from 7 to 67%, depending on the stringency of the diagnostic criteria and population studied.[3,4]

The main factors that lead to OSA in craniofacial syndromes appear to be midface and/or mandibular hypoplasia. These abnormalities impact not only the external appearance of the facial bone but also the UA internally. Moreover, such malformations may be part of syndromes that include neuromuscular disorders, resulting in poor pharyngeal neuromotor tone or other anatomic features such as macroglossia and glossoptosis that predispose to increased risk of UA collapse.[5]

Some of the treatment modalities are common to those used in otherwise healthy children with OSA (adenotonsillectomy, continuous positive airway pressure [CPAP]). However, because of the multifactorial cause of UA obstruction and because this is a heterogeneous and complex pediatric population, there are some distinct approaches to the management of children with craniofacial syndromes, such as insertion of nasopharyngeal airway and surgical interventions like midface advancement and mandibular distraction osteogenesis.[6]

Maxillofacial surgical intervention, by bypassing midface obstruction, can improve OSA in the majority of the cases, but many studies showed that respiratory outcome after maxillofacial surgery is not as successful as is generally thought, with about 30% of children showing no improvement of the sleep-disordered breathing (SDB).[7,8]

These results suggest that OSA, despite its strong correlationwith facial skeletal dysmorphology, is often a multilevel problem in these children, and treating it with maxillofacial surgery without further examination of its cause, might lead to under treatment or even mistreatment.[9]

22.1.1 Types of Craniofacial Diseases and OSA

See ▶ Table 22.1.

CFAs are uncommon conditions with heterogeneous phenotypes and may occur in isolation or as part of a syndrome. The Whitaker classification[10] separates CFAs into four groups, including a) clefts, b) synostoses, c) atrophy–hypoplasia, and d) neoplasia–hyperplasia, but there is no comprehensive system to classify all craniofacial conditions.

In children with syndromic craniofacial malformations, significant OSA may begin in the neonatal period, and

Table 22.1 Main causes of OSA in craniofacial conditions

Condition	Potential causes of OSAS
Cleft lip/palate	Nasal deformities, compensatory head position, short mandible
Hypoplasia	Micrognathia, glossoptosis, midface hypoplasia
Craniosynostosis	Midface hypoplasia, choanal atresia, palatal deformities

they were more likely to have a more severe condition than general pediatric population.

Because long-term sequelae of OSA in children are potentially serious, it is important to better understand the relationship between OSA and CFAs.

Furthermore, consideration of OSA diagnosis and treatment in children with CFA is particularly important because of the overlapping morbidity. Some craniofacial syndromes are associated with learning disabilities, neurocognitive deficits, or failure to thrive.[11] Because pediatric OSA also can result in these sequelae, it is possible that in children with CFA, these morbidities might be due, in part, to the associated OSA, which often can be treated. Thus, it appears especially important to identify and treat OSA in this subgroup of children.

22.1.2 Cleft Lip and/or Palate

See ▶ Fig. 22.1.

Cleft palate with or without a cleft lip is a relatively common birth defect, with an incidence of 0.69 to 2.51 per 1000 births worldwide. Epidemiological studies showed that approximately 70 to 80% of clefts occur in isolation, while the remaining are part of a syndrome or associated with other anomalies.

Syndromes that commonly include cleft palate include Pierre Robin sequence (PRS), Stickler syndrome, Treacher Collins syndrome (TCS), Goldenhar syndrome, and Nager syndrome.

In children with cleft lip/palate, the associated facial features include midface hypoplasia and a retrognathic maxilla, resulting in reduced UA dimensions and increased risk of OSA.

Approximately 34% of children with a syndromic diagnosis and 17% of nonsyndromic children are found to have OSA.[12]

In addition, OSA is also well-documented after surgical interventions to correct velopharyngeal incompetence.[13]

For these reasons, children with cleft palate should be carefully monitored for OSAS, especially after secondary palatoplasty.

22.1.3 Synostoses

Craniosynostoses are congenital conditions that include premature fusion of one or more of the cranial sutures, resulting in abnormal growth of the skull in the direction parallel to the fused suture. Craniosynostoses affect approximately one in 2500 live births and can be either syndromic or nonsyndromic. Common conditions that include craniosynostoses include Apert, Crouzon, and Pfeiffer syndromes.

Between 40 and 68% of children with syndromic craniosynostoses were found to have OSA, mainly due to midface hypoplasia, but other factors such as adenotonsillar hypertrophy, choanal atresia, palatal deformities, mandibular hypoplasia, and tracheal cartilage anomalies are also described as risk factors.[14]

22.1.4 Hypoplasia

Conditions that include midface and mandibular hypoplasia (▶ Fig. 22.2) are thought to cause OSA, due to obstruction at the base of the tongue from glossoptosis and reduced oropharyngeal airway size.

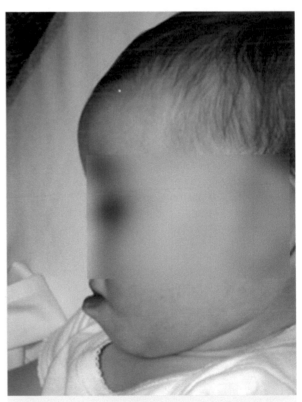

Fig. 22.2 A 1-year-old child suffering from midfacial hypoplasia associated with cleft lip and palate.

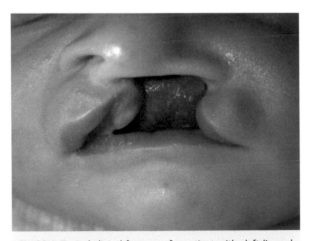

Fig. 22.1 Typical clinical features of a patient with cleft lip and palate.

PRS, a clinical anomaly characterized by mandibular hypoplasia, glossoptosis and a U-shaped cleft palate, is the most common cause of syndromic micrognathia.

TCS is a rare congenital craniofacial condition. Its deformities can range from a slight defect of the cilia to severe defects such as micrognathia and zygomatico-temporo–maxillary dysostosis. The main factor leading to OSA in TCS is mandibular hypoplasia.

The prevalence of OSA in children with PRS and TCS is 12.5% and 46%, respectively.[15]

Similar to PRS and TCS, patients with hemifacial microsomia (HM) have the potential for increased risk of OSA. HM includes malformations of the maxilla, mandible, temporomandibular joint, muscles of mastication, ear, and occasionally the facial nerve. Goldenhar syndrome is a variant of HM, with involvement of the eyes and spine.

A recent systematic review of the literature on children with HM showed prevalence of OSA ranging from 7 to 67%.[3]

22.2 Rationale for DISE in Children with Craniofacial Anomalies

See (▶ Table 22.2).

Over the past few years, attention has been drawn at identifying the site of UA obstruction in children with complex OSA as well as those with craniofacial malformations. Flexible fiberoptic endoscopy and cephalometry are the most commonly tools used to identify sites of UA obstruction in these children,[16] but they are limited by the fact that these evaluations are either static or performed during wakefulness, which may not accurately represent the dynamic UA collapse seen during sleep. To develop the most targeted and effective surgical treatment plan, drug-induced sleep endoscopy (DISE) has been developed to characterize the location and pattern of UA obstruction. For these patients, the paradigm of DISE-directed surgery, in which site(s) of anatomic airway obstruction are identified by DISE in order to guide treatment decision, may be an improvement from the existing surgical protocols.

Table 22.2 Surgical treatments for OSA in children with CFAs

Condition	Surgical treatment
Cleft lip/palate	Partial adenoidectomy, tonsillectomy
Hypoplasia	Mandibular distraction, midface advancement, lip adhesion, tracheotomy
Craniosynostosis	Midface advancement

Abbreviations: CFA, craniofacial anomalies; OSA, obstructive sleep apnea.

Nevertheless, there are a few studies focusing on the pediatric population with CFAs and evaluating the role of DISE in guiding directed decision treatment in this subgroup of children.

Myatt et al[17] reported on DISE findings in a heterogeneous group of 20 patients affected by OSA and obstructive awake apnea, looking into surgically naive syndromic and nonsyndromic children with complex and severe OSA.

The authors found that the site of airway obstruction varies in the individual child, even among children suffering from the same syndrome, thus explaining why some treatments for OSA may succeed in some children and fail in others.

The important conclusion regarding this study is that correction of the airway obstruction, targeted at the site of obstruction found on DISE, provided an excellent success rate with a decrease in the mean apnea–hypopnea index (AHI) from 48 to 4.6 per hour.

Finally, the authors advocate that DISE should be followed by rigid laryngobronchoscopic examination before embarking on corrective surgery, as distal airway abnormalities may be missed. Indeed, synchronous lower airway lesions, such as subglottic stenosis, tracheomalacia, innominate artery compression, bronchomalacia or vascular rings, have been identified in up to 27% of children with CFAs[18] (▶ Fig. 22.3).

Another study[19] investigated the role of DISE in children with Apert and Crouzon syndromes who were scheduled for midface advancement. Preoperatively, although midface hypoplasia was often present, the cause of UA obstruction in these patients was multilevel. Follow-up endoscopy, performed to evaluate the effect of

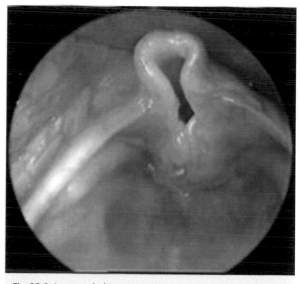

Fig. 22.3 Laryngeal obstruction due to ary-epiglottic folds collapse (DISE view). Abbreviation: DISE, drug-induced sleep endoscopy.

surgery, showed residual obstruction in all patients, not only at the level of the nose, but also frequently at the tongue base and hypopharynx.

These findings emphasized the importance of performing DISE before surgical intervention, since it can guide and optimize treatment in subjects suffering from OSA. As obstruction is usually present at multiple levels in the UA, midface hypoplasia is often not the only cause of OSA, and midface advancement may not successfully relieve the symptoms of airway obstruction if the levels of obstruction are not first identified.

Plompetalin a retrospective review of 11 children with TCS, who had moderate/severe OSA, reported various levels of obstruction from nose to trachea. In most of these patients, narrowing was present throughout the entire vertical pharyngeal height.[15] Overall, this is in contrast with these syndromic children, among whom midface hypoplasia with collapse at the level of the rhino–oropharynx is generally considered to be the major cause of obstruction.

In this series, five out of 11 patients who had midface advancement had persistent moderate-to-severe OSA requiring CPAP, and postoperative DISE revealed residual UA collapse with obstruction of the hypopharynx. The authors concluded that since OSA has a complex multiple level origin in TCS children, DISE is recommended to identify the exact levels of obstruction prior to maxillofacial dysmorphology surgical correction.

22.3 Conclusions

To date, the complexity of OSA in children with CFA is not fully recognized because of the multiple anatomical and systemic factors contributing to UA obstruction and because this is a heterogeneous and complex pediatric population. Most of the published literature on CFAs and sleep apnea is limited by including either individual case reports or retrospective reviews that encompass relatively small patient numbers. Conclusions from such studies are further hampered by the lack of objective data such as pre- and postoperative polysomnography (PSG) findings, lack of long-term outcomes and the heterogeneous phenotype of these patients, which dilutes the already scarce experience in the evaluation and management of single craniofacial conditions.

Although it was previously thought that OSA in these patients was strongly correlated to facial skeletal dysmorphology, recent studies have revealed that the etiology is often multifactorial, and the obstruction may occur anywhere along the UA (► Table 22.3). Multilevel obstruction (within both the upper and lower airway complexes) was observed between 40 and 67% of children with CFA.

Maxillofacial dismorphology correction can be effective in resolving airway obstruction, but in some cases, results have been somewhat less promising. Surgical treatment at one level is unlikely to resolve OSA due to its multilevel origin in this subgroup of patients. Although few data are

Table 22.3 Sites of obstruction on DISE in children with CFAs

Condition	DISE findings
Cleft lip/palate	Nasal obstruction, rhino-oropharynx obstruction
Hypoplasia	Rhinopharynx, tongue base and laryngohypopharynx obstruction
Craniosynostosis	Rhinopharynx, tongue base, and hypopharynx obstruction

Abbreviations: CFA, craniofacial anomalies; DISE, drug-induced sleep endoscopy.

available in literature, DISE seems to be a promising tool for UA evaluation and treatment selection in this subgroup of children. DISE may be recommended to identify the exact levels of obstruction and incorporate the findings in the treatment plan, providing a way to tailor better management for OSA in children with CFA. Finally, DISE should be followed by rigid laryngobronchoscopic examination before embarking on corrective surgery, as distal airway abnormalities may be missed.

References

[1] Alsubie HS, BaHammam AS. Obstructive sleep apnoea: children are not little adults. Paediatr Respir Rev. 2017; 21:72–79

[2] Tan HL, Kheirandish-Gozal L, Abel F, Gozal D. Craniofacial syndromes and sleep-related breathing disorders. Sleep Med Rev. 2016; 27: 74–88

[3] Caron CJ, Pluijmers BI, Joosten KF, et al. Obstructive sleep apnoea in craniofacial microsomia: a systematic review. Int J Oral Maxillofac Surg. 2015; 44(5):592–598

[4] Cielo CM, Marcus CL. Obstructive sleep apnoea in children with craniofacial syndromes. Paediatr Respir Rev. 2015; 16(3):189–196

[5] Garg RK, Afifi AM, Garland CB, Sanchez R, Mount DL. Pediatric obstructive sleep apnea: consensus, controversy, and craniofacial considerations. Plast Reconstr Surg. 2017; 140(5):987–997

[6] Sudarsan SS, Paramasivan VK, Arumugam SV, Murali S, Kameswaran M. Comparison of treatment modalities in syndromic children with obstructive sleep apnea–a randomized cohort study. Int J Pediatr Otorhinolaryngol. 2014; 78(9):1526–1533

[7] Moraleda-Cibrián M, Edwards SP, Kasten SJ, Buchman SR, Berger M, O'Brien LM. Obstructive sleep apnea pretreatment and posttreatment in symptomatic children with congenital craniofacial malformations. J Clin Sleep Med. 2015; 11(1):37–43

[8] Rosen D. Management of obstructive sleep apnea associated with Down syndrome and other craniofacial dysmorphologies. Curr Opin Pulm Med. 2011; 17(6):431–436

[9] Nout E, Bannink N, Koudstaal MJ, et al. Upper airway changes in syndromic craniosynostosis patients following midface or monobloc advancement: correlation between volume changes and respiratory outcome. J Craniomaxillofac Surg. 2012; 40(3):209–214

[10] Whitaker LA, Pashayan H, Reichman J. A proposed new classification of craniofacial anomalies. Cleft Palate J. 1981; 18(3):161–176

[11] Capdevila OS, Kheirandish-Gozal L, Dayyat E, Gozal D. Pediatric obstructive sleep apnea: complications, management, and long-term outcomes. Proc Am Thorac Soc. 2008; 5(2):274–282

[12] Muntz H, Wilson M, Park A, Smith M, Grimmer JF. Sleep disordered breathing and obstructive sleep apnea in the cleft population. Laryngoscope. 2008; 118(2):348–353

[13] Muntz HR. Management of sleep apnea in the cleft population. Curr Opin Otolaryngol Head Neck Surg. 2012; 20(6):518–521

[14] Driessen C, Joosten KF, Bannink N, et al. How does obstructive sleep apnoea evolve in syndromic craniosynostosis? A prospective cohort study. Arch Dis Child. 2013; 98(7):538–543

[15] Plomp RG, Bredero-Boelhouwer HH, Joosten KF, et al. Obstructive sleep apnoea in Treacher Collins syndrome: prevalence, severity and cause. Int J Oral Maxillofac Surg. 2012; 41(6):696–701

[16] Li KK, Guilleminault C, Riley RW, Powell NB. Obstructive sleep apnea and maxillomandibular advancement: an assessment of airway changes using radiographic and nasopharyngoscopic examinations. J Oral Maxillofac Surg. 2002; 60(5):526–530, discussion 531

[17] Myatt HM, Beckenham EJ. The use of diagnostic sleep nasendoscopy in the management of children with complex upper airway obstruction. Clin Otolaryngol Allied Sci. 2000; 25(3): 200–208

[18] de Jong T, Bannink N, Bredero-Boelhouwer HH, et al. Long-term functional outcome in 167 patients with syndromic craniosynostosis; defining a syndrome-specific risk profile. J Plast Reconstr Aesthet Surg. 2010; 63(10):1635–1641

[19] Doerga PN, Spruijt B, Mathijssen IM, Wolvius EB, Joosten KF, van der Schroeff MP. Upper airway endoscopy to optimize obstructive sleep apnea treatment in Apert and Crouzon syndromes. J Craniomaxillofac Surg. 2016; 44(2):191–196

23 Advanced Technique

Giovanni Sorrenti, Giuseppe Caccamo, Irene Pelligra, Luca Burgio, Riccardo Albertini, Eleonora Cioccoloni, Paolo Cozzolino, and Ottavio Piccin

Abstract

Predictors of treatment outcome are of primary importance for selecting suitable obstructive sleep apnea (OSA) patients who may benefit from nonventilatory therapeutic options. Compared with other methods of upper airway (UA) assessment, drug-induced sleep endoscopy (DISE) appears to be a promising technique to select the proper treatment for patients with OSA.

In this chapter, we describe an advanced technique of standardized DISE in which UA assessment is combined with polysomnographic monitoring and additional diagnostic maneuvers.

Keywords: obstructive sleep apnea, drug-induced sleep endoscopy, polysomnography, mandibular advancement device, upper airway assessment

23.1 Introduction

Currently, there is a wide range of treatment options for obstructive sleep apnea (OSA), including surgical interventions and noninvasive conservative measures. Among "nonventilatory" (non-PAP) conservative modalities, positional therapy (PT) and mandibular advancement devices (MADs) are the most offered options. MADs provide upper airway (UA) widening and reduction of the airway resistance, and are recommended by American Academy of Sleep Medicine and American Academy of Dental Sleep Medicine clinical practice guidelines, both as primary therapy and as an alternative approach for those patients unable to tolerate continuous positive airway pressure (CPAP).[1,2]

One of the factors limiting a successful response of non-PAP conservative treatments is the inability to identify those patients who will have a successful outcome prior to investing the time and resources necessary to implement this treatment. For this reason, predictors of treatment outcome are of primary importance for selecting suitable patients who might benefit from these alternative therapeutic options.

Compared to other methods of UA assessment, drug-induced sleep endoscopy (DISE) appears to be a useful tool to select the proper treatment for patients with OSA. The main advantage of DISE is to overcome the limit of awake endoscopy related to continuous neuromuscular control by the central nervous system that during sleep is physiologically decreased.[3,4]

One critical issue of DISE is the use of sedation and the possible effect of drugs on UA patency. Nevertheless, several studies have already proved the validity of DISE with target-controlled infusion (TCI) in reducing the probability of excessive muscle relaxation and accordingly false-positive obstructive events.[5,6]

Although interrater reliability and the test–retest reliability of DISE appear to be good,[7,8] another criticism of DISE is that the assessment of the UA is based on subjective observations. As a result, outcomes can vary by investigator's subjective interpretation of what they consider to be abnormal in the UA, so that DISE assessment could be imprecise in correlating UA collapse to respiratory events. Concerning what was just mentioned, "advanced" DISE (A-DISE) represents a technique to avoid these critical issues. It is a standardized DISE combined with simultaneous polysomnographic recording to evaluate the exact site and pattern of UA obstruction associated to respiratory events. Applying different passive tests, this technique provides important information on the dynamic changes of the UA patency and sleep parameters, in order to predict the possible benefit for different treatment options.

The aims of this chapter are to describe the steps of this technique and provide an overview of the potential advantages of A-DISE.

23.2 Indications

In our protocol, A-DISE is indicated to evaluate patients with moderate-to-severe OSA who have failed a trial of CPAP as first-line therapy, or patients with mild OSA without cardiovascular comorbidities who prefer alternative treatments before committing to lifelong CPAP use.

23.2.1 Assessment before A-DISE

A comprehensive ENT clinically based evaluation, including awake video endoscopy with Müller maneuver and lateral cephalometry, is done before the procedure.

The diagnosis of OSA is based on the 8-channel home sleep apnea test (HSAT, type III polygraphy; Embletta Gold, Embla System Inc). Sleep recordings are always scored manually in a standard fashion by board-certified sleep professionals, according to the AASM Manual for the Scoring of Sleep and Associated Events Rules, Terminology and Technical Specification.[9]

23.2.2 Titration Approach for Oral Device Simulator

The procedure is preceded by the registration of a specific simulation bite, custom-made for each patient. The

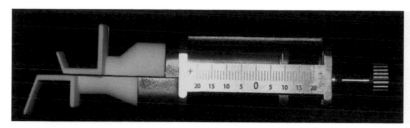

Fig. 23.1 The sliding caliper and simulation bite.

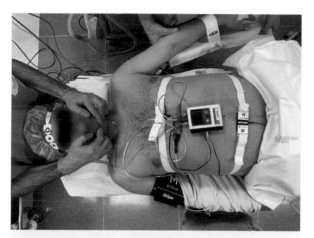

Fig. 23.2 A typical set up in operating room during A-DISE. Abbreviation: DISE, drug-induced sleep endoscopy.

orthodontist performs a comprehensive assessment of the patient (dental, periodontal, and functional examination) and uses a dedicated registration fork to set the anterior bite opening and the likely initial therapeutic protrusion for future MAD fitting.

First, the upper arch of the fork is covered with a registration material (hard putty silicone) and left to cure once placed against the upper jaw.

The patient is then asked to protrude the mandible maximally, followed by a slow retraction, until a position is reached that the patient described as the maximal comfortable protrusive position (generally 70% of the maximal protrusion).

This position is then recorded with the lower arch of the fork covered with the same bite-registration material, resulting in the simulation bite ready to be used during DISE. Finally, the simulation bite is placed on a sliding caliper with a tethered locking mechanism, providing 1-millimeter adjustments across protrusive ranges (▶ Fig. 23.1).

23.2.3 A-DISE Protocol

DISE is performed in a semi-dark and silent operating room (OR), with the patient lying in the supine position on an operating table. Prior to the IV administration of the sedative drugs, the simulation bite is positioned

intraorally, in order to avoid waking up the patient, and electrodes, wires and sensors to record sleep parameters are placed (▶ Fig. 23.2). Artificial sleep is induced by IV administration of propofol through TCI (the initial infusion rate of propofol is 50 to 75 µg/kg/min). TCI is implemented with a syringe infusion pump, using the pharmacokinetic modeling program Stanpump and the Marsh weight-adjusted kinetic set for propofol. Sedation level is monitored using bispectral index monitor (BIS). Once the patient has reached a satisfactory level of sedation (BIS level between 50 and 70), a high-resolution flexible nasopharyngoscope, connected with a digital camera and high-resolution video monitor, is passed through the nose for inspection of the entire UA.

The endoscopic video recording is included in the sleep file as a video of the video-EEG system. In this way, both devices are perfectly synchronized for capturing and visualizing endoscopic and polysomnographic data simultaneously in real-time (▶ Fig. 23.3 and **Video 10**).

UA collapsibility and simultaneous polysomnographic recording with the simulation bite *in situ* are examined during at least two or more respiratory cycles, consisting of a stable and complete sequence of snoring, obstructive hypopnea/apnea, oxygen desaturation and rebreathing for all the UA levels.

Afterward, the simulation bite is progressively advanced in 1 mm increment until snoring, apneas and hypopneas are eliminated, and UA collapse is partially or completely resolved. This phase of DISE allows easy determination of an efficacious jaw position which can be transferred to the custom oral device. When UA collapse is partially or completely resolved and PSG parameters are normal, the patient may be considered an excellent suitable candidate for MAD treatment (▶ Fig. 23.4).

The concept is analogous to polysomnography (PSG) with CPAP titration, which is performed prior to initiating patients on CPAP treatment in order to identify the optimal pressure setting and demonstrate an acceptable reduction in apnea–hypopnea index (AHI).

After this phase of DISE, the simulation bite is removed, and the endoscopic findings and polysomnographic data are observed in a normal baseline setting without any mandibular protrusion effect (▶ Fig. 23.5).

To assess the influence of head and body position on UA obstruction and polysomnographic recordings, DISE is carried out during head and trunk rotation. This maneuver can be particularly important for positional OSA

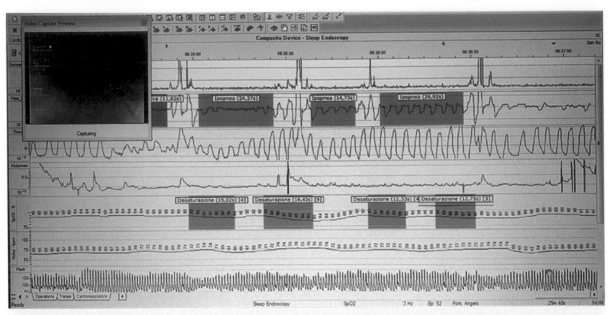

Fig. 23.3 The endoscopic video recording included in the PSG file for capturing and visualizing UA and polysomnographic data simultaneously in real-time. Abbreviations: PSG, polysomnography; UA, upper airway.

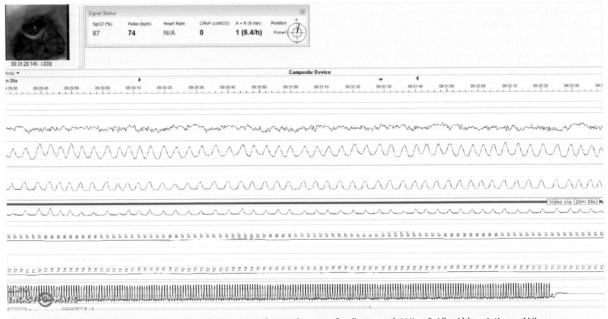

Fig. 23.4 Endoscopic UA evaluation with oral device simulator: absence of collapse and AHI = 6.4/h. Abbreviations: AHI, apnea–hypopnea index; UA, upper airway.

patients when incorporation of PT in the treatment plan is considered. The improvement of UA collapse and respiratory events during head and/or trunk rotation can be considered a predictive positive factor for treatment response to PT.

The final step consists of "transoral" DISE to evaluate the tongue–palate interaction which is difficult to detect while looking at the airway from behind (see **Video 10**).

During transoral DISE, the fiber endoscope is smoothly pushed between the upper and lower incisors with no

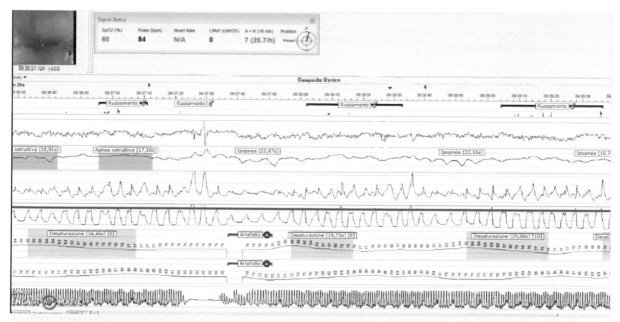

Fig. 23.5 Baseline endoscopic UA Evaluation: Complete anteroposterior palatal collapse of the UA and AHI = 25.7/h. Abbreviations: AHI, apnea–hypopnea index; UA, upper airway.

need to open the mouth in order to avoid the effect of mouth breathing on UA structures. When the dorsum of the tongue is attached to the soft palate, and together with it moves backward, occluding the airway, the retro-palatal obstruction is secondary to posterior displacement of the tongue. In these patients, the objective of correction should be the tongue and not the soft palate.

Both endoscopic and polysomnographic recordings are collected for later offline review. The total amount duration of this procedure is about 20 to 25 minutes.

23.3 Potential Advantages from Conventional Technique

Identifying OSA patients who are likely to be successful treatment candidates would be desirable from both therapeutic and financial perspectives. The inability to prospectively identify patients who will experience therapeutic success continues to limit the clinical utility of non-PAP therapies. In this context, the main role of DISE is to help determine the treatment modality tailored for each individual patient.

Concerning MADs, several studies have reported that awake video-endoscopy of the UA is a useful method of achieving good effectiveness for oral appliances treatment, because it allows the clinician to decide the appropriate mandibular position by directly evaluating the changes in the airway patency with mandibular protrusion.[10,11] Other authors showed a significant association between the findings during DISE with manual jaw advancement or

simulation bite and treatment response with oral devices.[12,13] It is well-established that mandibular protrusion has a dose-dependent effect on the pharyngeal cross-sectional area. More protrusion of the mandible leads to larger improvements in OSA.[14,15] However, excessive mandibular protrusion may lead to temporo-mandibular disturbances, tooth pain and movements of the teeth.

A-DISE, through the simultaneous evaluation of changes both in UA patency and polysomnographic data, allows to determine the efficacy of mandibular advancement in controlling respiratory events, providing a reliable estimate of the minimum displacement of advancement to treat sleep apnea.

The identification of the minimum therapeutic protrusion level by this method may help in reducing side effects produced by further unnecessary titration and improving adherence.

Focusing on positional OSA, the evaluation of UA patency and polysomnographic recording in different sleep positions, may identify patients who can effectively benefit from PT.

Definitely, A-DISE can provide data to use in prospective decision-making in the individual patient, in order to not only improve the clinical effectiveness of the treatment but also help prevent unrealistic expectations regarding the available treatment for each patient.

In conclusion, A-DISE, providing simultaneous evaluation of UA obstruction and respiratory events during induced sleep, has the potential to be a reliable approach to select a "tailored therapy" for each patient. One of the disadvantages is that this technique is resource-intensive, requiring the otolaryngologist, anesthesiologist, orthodontist and sleep technician as well as advanced equipment and more time than usual.

References

[1] Kushida CA, Morgenthaler TI, Littner MR, et al. American Academy of Sleep. Practice parameters for the treatment of snoring and obstructive sleep apnea with oral appliances: an update for 2005. Sleep. 2006; 29(2):240–243

[2] Ramar K, Dort LC, Katz SG, et al. Clinical practice guideline for the treatment of obstructive sleep apnea and snoring with oral appliance therapy: an update for 2015. J Clin Sleep Med. 2015; 11(7): 773–827

[3] Certal VF, Pratas R, Guimarães L, et al. Awake examination versus DISE for surgical decision making in patients with OSA: a systematic review. Laryngoscope. 2016; 126(3):768–774

[4] Zerpa Zerpa V, Carrasco Llatas M, Agostini Porras G, Dalmau Galofre J. Drug-induced sedation endoscopy versus clinical exploration for the diagnosis of severe upper airway obstruction in OSAHS patients. Sleep Breath. 2015; 19(4):1367–1372

[5] De Vito A, Carrasco Llatas M, Vanni A, et al. European position paper on drug-induced sedation endoscopy (DISE). Sleep Breath. 2014; 18 (3):453–465

[6] De Vito A, Carrasco Llatas M, Ravesloot MJ, et al. European position paper on drug-induced sleep endoscopy: 2017 Update. Clin Otolaryngol. 2018; 43(6):1541–1552

[7] Kezirian EJ, White DP, Malhotra A, Ma W, McCulloch CE, Goldberg AN. Interrater reliability of drug-induced sleep endoscopy. Arch Otolaryngol Head Neck Surg. 2010; 136(4):393–397

[8] Golbin D, Musgrave B, Succar E, Yaremchuk K. Clinical analysis of drug-induced sleep endoscopy for the OSA patient. Laryngoscope. 2016; 126(1):249–253

[9] International Classification of Sleep Disorders: Diagnostic and Coding Manual. 2nd ed. Westchester: American Academy of Sleep Medicine; 2005

[10] Sasao Y, Nohara K, Okuno K, Nakamura Y, Sakai T. Videoendoscopic diagnosis for predicting the response to oral appliance therapy in severe obstructive sleep apnea. Sleep Breath. 2014; 18(4):809–815

[11] Okuno K, Sasao Y, Nohara K, et al. Endoscopy evaluation to predict oral appliance outcomes in obstructive sleep apnoea. Eur Respir J. 2016; 47(5):1410–1419

[12] Johal A, Battagel JM, Kotecha BT. Sleep nasendoscopy: a diagnostic tool for predicting treatment success with mandibular advancement splints in obstructive sleep apnoea. Eur J Orthod. 2005; 27(6): 607–614

[13] Vanderveken OM, Vroegop AVM, Van de Heyning PH, Braem MJ. Drug-induced sleep endoscopy completed with a simulation bite approach for the prediction of the outcome of treatment of obstructive sleep apnea with mandibular repositioning appliances. Oper Tech Otolaryngol. 2011; 22:175–182

[14] Zhang M, Liu Y, Liu Y, et al. Effectiveness of oral appliances versus continuous positive airway pressure in treatment of OSA patients: an updated meta-analysis. Cranio. 2018; 24:1–18

[15] Bonetti GA, Piccin O, Lancellotti L, Bianchi A, Marchetti C. A case report on the efficacy of transverse expansion in severe obstructive sleep apnea syndrome. Sleep Breath. 2009; 13(1):93–96

24 Future Perspectives

A. Simon Carney, Peter Catcheside, and Alex Wall

Abstract

While drug-induced sleep endoscopy (DISE) continues to establish itself in surgical treatment algorithms, it has notable limitations. In particular, it cannot faithfully recreate the sleep stages now well-recognized to influence the behavior of the pharyngeal musculature. This varies markedly between rapid eye movement (REM) and over the course of deepening non-REM sleep, changing muscle tone and arousal propensity. Recent research efforts have identified complementary, noninvasive methods of upper airway (UA) assessment to try and identify the role, site and magnitude of anatomical collapse during all sleep phases in patients with obstructive sleep apnea (OSA). These techniques include patient phenotyping/endotyping techniques designed to better understand anatomical and nonanatomical causal factors on an individual patient basis, analysis of airflow shape, radiological sleep analysis, and real-time sleep videomanometry. These newer experimental techniques are still in their infancy and at this stage are not considered as a replacement for DISE. However, these emerging methods are likely to add to our future armamentarium for the analysis of site or sites of airway collapse, role of neuromuscular and respiratory control, and arousal factors in the complex pathophysiology of OSA.

Keywords: recent advances, videomanometry, cine MRI, sleep MRI, airflow shape, phenotyping, endotyping

24.1 Patient Phenotyping/Endotyping

It is now recognized that obstructive sleep apnea (OSA) is a heterogeneous disorder for which a "one size fits all" treatment approach fails to successfully treat many patients.[1] Strong evidence now supports that there are at least four main traits ("endotypes" or "phenotypes") that contribute to the propensity for, and severity of, airway collapse during sleep (▶ Fig. 24.1). While a narrow and/or collapsible airway remains the key problem for the majority of patients, nonanatomical factors such as poor airway dilator muscle function, unstable respiratory control ("high-loop gain"), and a low respiratory arousal threshold can play an important part in the etiology of OSA.[1] Identification of the presence and magnitude of these nonanatomical factors are likely to help determine which patients are likely to do well with upper airway (UA) surgery, and more importantly, to identify patients more likely to get a poor result and for whom other treatment modalities would be more preferable.[1]

24.1.1 Deficient Upper Airway Anatomy

There is no doubt that a narrow and/or collapsible UA is the key cause of OSA in most patients.[1] Continuous positive airway pressure (CPAP), dental devices and multilevel sleep surgery are all directed at resolving this very problem.[2] Obesity contributes to airway collapse via increased fat deposition in the neck, pharyngeal muscles, the tongue and abdomen, all of which may influence airway function via airway crowding, mass loading, and reduced caudal tracheal traction effects. There is also evidence that the stiffness of the tongue is lower in patients with OSA.

Whilst awake UA examination techniques such as Müller's maneuver and Woodson's hypotonic method can help to identify the site and degree of collapsibility while a patient is awake,[2] new techniques now allow for the assessment of degree of collapse during sleep.

The passive critical closing pressure (Pcrit) of the airway identifies the pressure required to achieve total airway collapse during sleep. A patient wears a modified CPAP device that can deliver both positive and negative

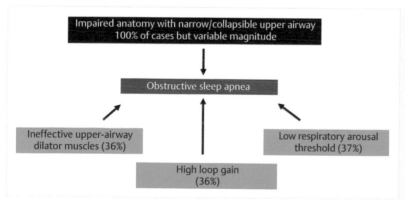

Fig. 24.1 Schematic diagram of the four main endotypes/phenotypes contributing to OSA. Abbreviation: OSA, obstructive sleep apnea.

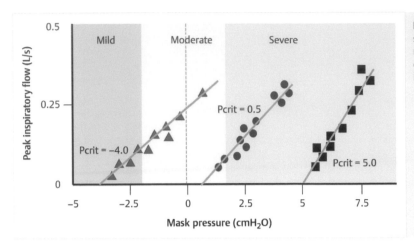

Fig. 24.2 Measurement of Pcrit. This figure shows three examples of Pcrit where multiple reductions in pressure have been obtained. The point at which the regression line crosses the X-axis is the Pcrit.

pressure. After maintaining the airway with positive pressure to maintain a fully open airway with relatively low breathing drive (and thus largely passive UA muscle activity), the pressure is then abruptly lowered during brief pressure drops that typically last at least five breaths. This procedure is typically performed during nonrapid eye movement (REM) sleep and is designed to induce different severities of partial airway collapse and airflow limitation, using variable positive and negative pressures as required. From multiple pressure drops over the night, a plot of average peak inspiratory flow versus end-expiratory mask pressure can be plotted. Extrapolation of the line to where it crosses the X-axis (i.e., with zero flow) identifies the Pcrit. Patients without OSA (or very mild airway collapse) classically show Pcrit <−2.0 cmH_2O. Moderately collapsible airways are defined as being near to atmospheric pressure, where Pcrit is between −2.0 and +2.0 cmH_2O and severely collapsible airways above 2.0 cmH_2O, indicating an airway that requires more substantial pressure to maintain patency (▶ Fig. 24.2).

24.1.2 Muscle Responsiveness

The pharyngeal airway is a complex muscular tube which substantially relies on central neural mechanisms to maintain its patency.[1] The gravitational effect of surrounding tissues and dynamic negative intraluminal pressure forces acting on the airway throughout each breathing cycle. Genioglossus and tensor veli palatini are the two main muscular dilator muscles and are activated via neural reflex loops in response to respiration and, importantly, changing airway pressure and collapse during sleep. In a normal airway, genioglossus activity abruptly decreases at sleep onset, followed by a compensatory increase to above wake levels throughout N2 to slow wave sleep.[1] Tonic muscles such as tensor palatini behave quite differently and typically show abrupt decrease at sleep onset and throughout sleep. All muscles show quite

profound hypotonia in REM sleep, thus explaining why OSA are most severe during this sleep phase. During airway obstruction, a rise in CO_2 and airway pressure changes contribute to increased dilator muscle activity, termed "muscle responsiveness," which varies across individuals. In over 33% of patient with OSA, genioglossus muscle responsiveness is low or absent. In others, muscle responsiveness is preserved during non-REM sleep (which protects the airway in patients with anatomical compromise and Pcrit <−5 cmH_2O) but reduces in REM sleep, leading to insufficient dilatory activity and maintaining airway patency in patients with impaired anatomy and a low Pcrit.

24.1.3 Loop Gain

The main driver of breathing during sleep is a rise in CO_2, and CO_2 chemosensitivity varies between individuals. High-CO_2 sensitivity promotes unstable control which can contribute to oscillations in breathing in both central and OSA. The sensitivity of the ventilatory control system is well-characterized by the concept of "loop gain," which is the ratio of the magnitude of the control system response to a ventilatory disturbance relative to the disturbance itself. Patients with a high-loop gain exhibit excessive changes in breathing in response to relatively small changes in CO_2. A diagrammatic representation of high-loop gain is shown in ▶ Fig. 24.3.

Exaggerated ventilatory oscillations with high-loop gain promote unstable ventilatory overshoot and undershoot responses promoting airway collapse and cyclical hypopnea/apnea. Over 33% of OSA patients demonstrate high-loop gain (defined in that particular study as 5 L/min increase to a normal 1 L/min stimulus).[1]

A retrospective analysis of patients who underwent multilevel UA surgery for sleep apnea demonstrated that patients with a lower loop gain achieved better outcomes from surgery than those with higher loop gain.[3] While this does not necessarily mean that the patients with

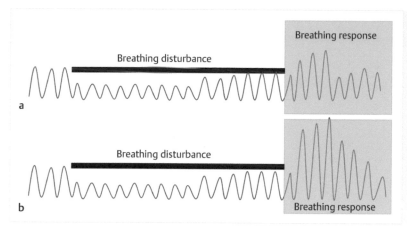

Fig. 24.3 Schematic representation of low (a) versus high (b) loop gain. After normal breathing, a reduction in CPAP occurs, creating a breathing disturbance. When breathing is restored, in **a**, a slight increase occurs before settling back to steady state within a few breaths. In **b**, breathing peaks of much higher magnitude are seen, taking longer to settle back to steady state normal breathing. Abbreviation: CPAP, continuous positive airway pressure.

higher loop gain should be denied surgical intervention, it is one of several parameters that may be useful in a multidisciplinary setting toward identifying patients with low-loop gain who are more likely to gain benefit from surgery and those with a higher loop gain for whom a successful surgical outcome may be unlikely.[4] This will allow for better patient consent and discussion and optimize patient outcomes.

24.1.4 Respiratory Arousal Threshold

It was previously thought that cortical arousals were essential to restore airflow after a respiratory event in patients with OSA. However, approximately 20% of respiratory events in adults terminate without arousal.[1] This is even higher in children (50%) and infants (>90%). In contrast, approximately 20% of arousals occur after complete airflow recovery, further highlighting the independent nature of arousal and airflow recovery in many cases. The level of inspiratory effort associated with respiratory-related arousal is termed the "respiratory arousal threshold." Especially in nonobese patients with OSA, between 30 to 50% of patients show arousal to relatively small changes in negative intrathoracic pressure (i.e., a low-respiratory arousal threshold). In slow wave sleep, the respiratory arousal threshold is higher, which likely promotes higher inspiratory and UA dilator muscle activity; this allows most patients with OSA who can achieve deep slow wave sleep demonstrate fewer respiratory events. However, in individuals with a low-respiratory arousal threshold, frequent arousals can delay and even prevent progression to deeper and more stable stages of sleep.[1]

24.1.5 PALM Scale for Patient Phenotyping

The PALM (<u>P</u>crit, <u>a</u>rousal threshold, <u>l</u>oop gain and <u>m</u>uscle responsiveness) scale has been developed toward classifying patients into groups in order to help better direct therapy to underlying physiological deficits.[1] Groups are identified according to the levels of Pcrit. PALM 1 (Pcrit >+2 cmH$_2$O) patients have severe anatomical collapse, PALM 2 (Pcrit −2.0 − +2.0 cmH$_2$O), moderate, and PALM 3 (Pcrit <2.0 cmH$_2$O) only minor anatomical problems. As PALM 2 comprises the largest group, this can be subdivided into PALM 2a where there is NO evidence of nonanatomical phenotype and PALM 2b where individuals have one or more "ALM" features. In a cohort of 54 patients assessed using the PALM criteria, the distribution of patients was as shown in ► Fig. 24.4.

24.1.6 Phenotyping/Endotyping Conclusions

Patient phenotyping/endotyping is an exciting area of future development. It highlights the need for multidisciplinary input into the identification of patients most suitable for UA surgery[2] (or other alternative OSA treatments) when CPAP fails or is not tolerated (► Fig. 24.5).

24.2 Analysis of Airflow Shape

Patients with obstructive sleep apnea frequently show narrowing or collapse of one or more anatomical areas.[2] During DISE, most observers would be aware that the pattern of obstruction varies from one individual to another. During airway collapse, the pattern of airflow reduction can be observed during natural sleep using simultaneous nasal and pharyngeal pressure recordings. In a recent study from the Harvard Medical School,[5] 31 subjects with sleep apnea were assessed using airflow and pharyngeal pressure measurements and simultaneous sleep video with a pediatric fiber optic endoscope placed in the postnasal space. The researchers were able to identify different patterns of inspiratory flow and negative effort dependence with reduced airflow despite increased respiratory effort, depending on whether the area of collapse was located in the retrolingual segment,

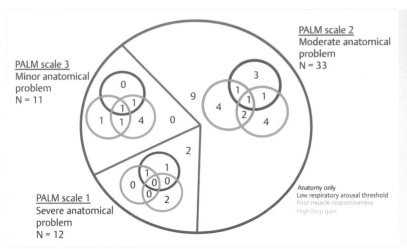

Fig. 24.4 A Venn diagram showing the overlap of the various OSA phenotypes in a study of 54 patients categorized into PALM scale. Abbreviation: OSA, obstructive sleep apnea.

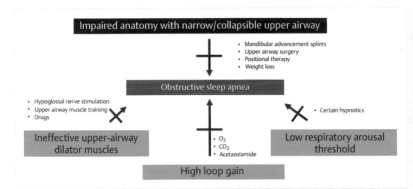

Fig. 24.5 Treatment methods applicable to OSA phenotypes. Abbreviation: OSA, obstructive sleep apnea.

retropalatal segment or with lateral wall collapse. Perhaps even more importantly, very clear identification of epiglottic collapse was also possible.[5]

With epiglottic collapse, a sudden obstruction of the airway with almost complete discontinuity of airflow was observed. During nonobstructed breaths, airflow continued as normal. With retrolingual obstruction, a flattened airflow pattern was observed. With palatal obstruction, a large movement of the palate coincided with moderate negative effort dependence (► Fig. 24.6 and ► Fig. 24.7).

It is not yet clear how important single versus multilevel collapse contributed to these important pioneering findings. While the airflow patterns discovered in this paper may not yet be immediately translatable into routine clinical practice, they provide an important benchmark for future research in this area (see real-time sleep videomanometry at the end of this chapter).

24.3 Radiological Sleep Assessment

Radiological assessment of the airway in patients with sleep apnea is not new. Standard airway cephalometry using either plain X-rays or computed tomography (CT) have long been used as a screening tool for surgery.[6] Several tests have been modified to be applicable to patients during sedated sleep. These include fluoroscopy, ultrafast CT and cine magnetic resonance imaging (MRI). The increased speed of MRI has proved attractive in that it is potentially suitable to assess the airway in real-time during natural or sedated sleep.[7] It is not without its challenges as MRI occurs in a noisy environment and can produce claustrophobia due to the narrow entry into the gantry tube. MRI is also relatively expensive. Nevertheless, early work using cineMRI (often termed sleep MRI in the literature) has shown interesting results in both adult[8] and paediatric[9] settings (► Fig. 24.8).

In adults, the availability of 3 Tesla MRI has greatly increased the resolution of sleep images.[7] In a study of 30 patients with mild–severe OSA,[8] sleep MRI was able to identify airway collapse in three sites (retropalatal, retrolingual and lateral pharyngeal wall). The 15 patients with severe OSA all had multilevel collapse with all three segments obstructing in 40% of cases, and retropalatal and lateral wall regions in the remaining 60%, The 15 patients with only mild OSA all demonstrated retropalatal collapse which was isolated to this single site in 80% of cases.

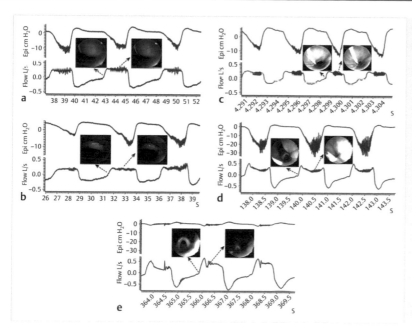

Fig. 24.6 Representation of flow shape and endoscopic images at different stage of respiration. (**a, b**) Velopharynx (**a**) and oropharynx (**b**) views of the same patient demonstrating retrolingual collapse. (**c, d**) Isolated retropalatal (**c**) and lateral wall (**d**) collapse in separate patients. (**e**) Epiglottic collapse with large and abrupt airflow changes. (From Genta PR et al. Airflow Shape is Associated with the Pharyngeal Structure Causing OSA. *Chest.* 2017, with permission).

The remaining mild OSA cases had retropalatal and retrolingual collapse in 13%, and retropalatal and lateral wall collapse in 7%.

In children, cineMRI has been used to good effect in patients with Down syndrome, demonstrating the quantity and degree of obstruction from lingual tonsil tissue in patients with persistent sleep apnea after adenotonsillectomy.[9] While cineMRI remains a new and relatively experimental technique, it can potentially play a role in more complex patients with sleep apnea. As MRI techniques become quieter, it may evolve into a more established and helpful investigative methodology in the future.

Criticisms of sleep MRI are that it remains noisy and sound-cancelling ear buds need to be used to help allow sleep. It can only be performed in the supine position, and simultaneous assessment of sleep-stage is difficult due to the magnetic field effects on conventional EEG leads. It is likely that sleep MRI only captures either stage 1 or stage 2 (NREM) sleep and may therefore not provide the REM data of most relevance for OSA assessment.[8]

Because of the relative limitations of cine MRI, more noninvasive assessment techniques of the airway during natural sleep have been attempted. A recent study from South Korea attached surface fiducial landmarks (that were meant to correlate to palatal and tongue position, confirmed with MRI) and monitored them with surface electrical impedance tomography (EIT) during natural sleep.[10] The authors claim EIT (in a pilot study of seven controls and 10 patients with OSA) provided successful identification of the site of airway closure in all patients with sleep apnea. No significant changes in the EIT data were observed in the seven control patients. As scientific advances may allow for the relatively stable positioning of electrodes both on the surface and within the tongue and palate, these sorts of methods of airway assessment may well evolve in the future and could well be an area of interest.

24.4 Real-Time Sleep Videomanometry

The use of airway manometry during natural sleep is again not a new concept. The apneagraph was a 2-electrode manometry catheter used to try and identify pressure changes in the UA in both the retropalatal and retrolingual segment.[11] Although initial results were encouraging, accidental movement of the manometry catheter distorted results and the apneagraphs failed to translate into routine clinical practice. While many observers initially expressed concerns that the presence of a manometry catheter could alter sleep and airway behavior parameters, analysis of polysomnography (PSG) results both with and without a manometry catheter in place are reassuringly unchanged.[12] As such, more advanced manometry analysis is a potential source of noninvasive airway assessment for the future.

With advances in fiber optic technology, it is now possible to construct thin catheters with pressure and temperature sensors every centimeter. In addition, the development of small "rice grain" micro charge-coupled device (CCD) video cameras also allows the potential for real-time airway visualization during natural sleep.[13]

A high-resolution, multichannel fiber optic CCT videomanometer is currently undergoing clinical evaluation in

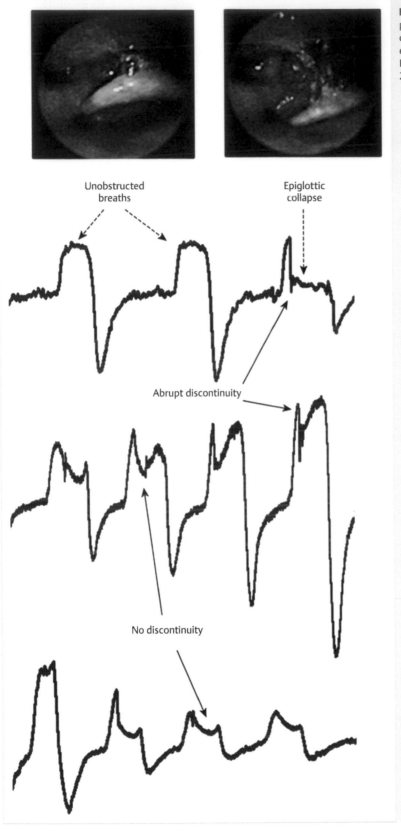

Fig. 24.7 Epiglottic collapse in different patients demonstrating sudden abrupt discontinuity of airflow (From Genta PR et al. Airflow Shape is Associated with the Pharyngeal Structure Causing OSA. *Chest*. 2017, with permission).

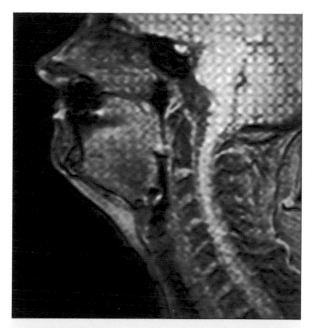

Fig. 24.8 Sleep MRI demonstrating retropalatal collapse (Image courtesy of Dr Lynne Bilston). Abbreviation: MRI, magnetic resonance imaging.

Australia. The catheter features a series of 12 equally spaced fiber optic pressure sensors and a micro camera mounted at the proximal end of the catheters' sensing region (▶ Fig. 24.9).

The camera body and wire has been integrated within the catheter silicone lumen to minimize any external protrusion, creating a flexible sealed unit. Illumination is provided from an LED and driver via a multimode fiber from within the translucent lumen (▶ Fig. 24.10).

Utilizing fiber Bragg grating (FBG) technology and a patented wavelength-division multiplexed helical sensor concept, the fiber optic array is being optimized for the requirements of the UA pressure measurements.[13] This configuration provides the ability to distinguish between pressure and temperature when both variables change at the same time over each breathing cycle. Pressure will accurately locate the point(s) of collapse within the soft UA while contact force via electrical impedance, along with changes in temperature swings at each sensing site, will help to give an indication of the severity of collapse and airflow reduction. Once the site of collapse has been identified, the micro video camera will identify the anatomical features and patterns of collapse involved.

Pilot studies have demonstrated that the pressure recordings seen in the fiber optic pressure waveforms

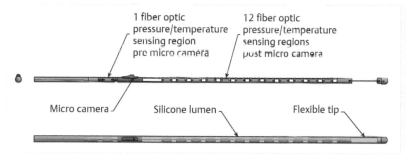

Fig. 24.9 High resolution videomanometry catheter. The camera body and wire has been integrated within the silicone sheath lumen to minimize any external protrusion and create a flexible sealed unit. Illumination is provided from an LED and driver via a multimode fiber from within the translucent lumen.

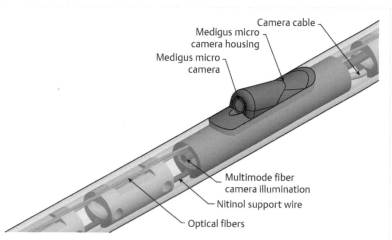

Fig. 24.10 Utilizing FBG technology and a patented wavelength-division multiplexed helical sensor concept, the fiber optic array is being optimized for the requirements of the UA application. This allows for the detection of pressure and temperature at the same time. Temperature swings can quantify residual flow past areas of partial occlusion or identify cessation of flow in the event of total occlusion. The video camera can identify the anatomical site and nature of the collapse. Abbreviations: FBG, fiber Bragg grafting; UA, upper airway.

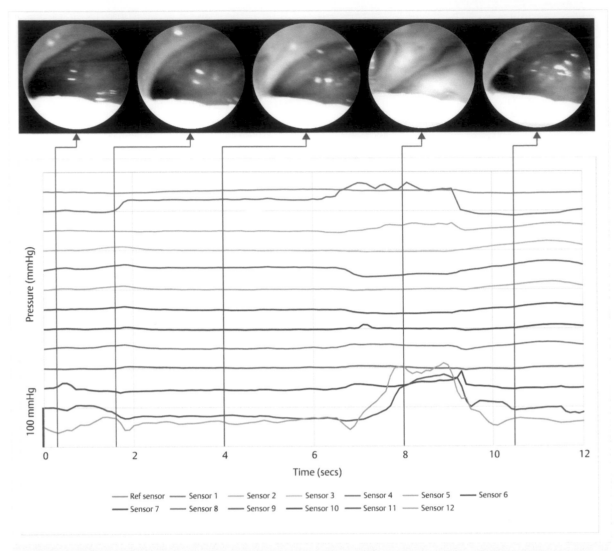

Fig. 24.11 Video camera images and pressure measurements during a retropalatal collapse. The lower electrodes are also detecting a probable simultaneous retrolingual collapse which could be identified by advancing the camera below the palatal obstruction.

correlate well to site of airway obstruction (▶ Fig. 24.11). These obstructive episodes can be anatomically confirmed with the video camera.[13]

The videomanometer is still in prototype development and design challenges faced to date include occlusion of the video image by nasal and pharyngeal secretions, LED light used to illuminate the airway causing sleep disruption, and accidental rotation of the catheter at night, providing poor imaging of the airway. Ongoing research is likely to overcome the majority of these issues, so that repositioning of the catheter by a well-trained sleep technician should reduce these problems during PSG. The advantage of a videomanometer analysis is that it can occur during natural sleep and at the same time as PSG. This would potentially provide the multidisciplinary sleep team with important new information regarding the site and degree of airway collapse to assist with predicting not only which patients might be more suitable for primary surgical management, but also which of the many surgical options are most likely to benefit any particular patient.[2]

24.5 Conclusions

While DISE can provide important information regarding the site and degree of airway collapse, the cost of the technique, requirement for access to an operating theatre environment, and concerns about the applicability of sedation findings to the most relevant phases of natural sleep have driven an ongoing search for more noninvasive methods which identify site-of-collapse in a more natural sleep setting. Further research in this area shows significant promise but outcome data will need to be compared to treatment outcome data based on the findings of DISE, which is the current main clinical technique for analysis of airway site-of-collapse.

References

[1] Eckert DJ. Phenotypic approaches to obstructive sleep apnoea: new pathways for targeted therapy. Sleep Med Rev. 2018; 37:45–59

[2] Carney AS, Antic NA, Catcheside PG, et al. Sleep Apnea Multilevel Surgery (SAMS) trial protocol: a multicenter randomized clinical trial of upper airway surgery for patients with obstructive sleep apnea who have failed continuous positive airway pressure. Sleep (Basel). 2019; 42(6):4

[3] Joosten SA, Leong P, Landry SA, et al. Loop gain predicts the response to upper airway surgery in patients with obstructive sleep apnea. Sleep (Basel). 2017; 40(7):1

[4] Hobson JC, Robinson S, Antic NA, et al. What is "success" following surgery for obstructive sleep apnea? The effect of different polysomnographic scoring systems. Laryngoscope. 2012; 122(8):1878–1881

[5] Genta PR, Sands SA, Butler JP, et al. Airflow shape is associated with the pharyngeal structure causing OSA. Chest. 2017; 152(3):537–546

[6] Chen W, Gillett E, Khoo MCK, Davidson Ward SL, Nayak KS. Real-time multislice MRI during continuous positive airway pressure reveals upper airway response to pressure change. J Magn Reson Imaging. 2017; 46(5):1400–1408

[7] Shin LK, Holbrook AB, Capasso R, et al. Improved sleep MRI at 3 tesla in patients with obstructive sleep apnea. J Magn Reson Imaging. 2013; 38(5):1261–1266

[8] Brown E, Bilston L. Case study: imaging of apnea termination in a patient with obstructive sleep apnea during natural sleep. J Clin Sleep Med. 2016; 12(11):1563–1564

[9] Ishman SL, Chang KW, Kennedy AA. Techniques for evaluation and management of tongue-base obstruction in pediatric obstructive sleep apnea. Curr Opin Otolaryngol Head Neck Surg. 2018; 26(6):409–416

[10] Kim YE, Woo EJ, Oh TI, Kim SW. Real-time identification of upper airway occlusion using electrical impedance tomography. J Clin Sleep Med. 2019; 15(4):563–571

[11] Morales Divo C, Selivanova O, Mewes T, Gosepath J, Lippold R, Mann WJ. Polysomnography and ApneaGraph in patients with sleep-related breathing disorders. ORL J Otorhinolaryngol Relat Spec. 2009; 71(1):27–31

[12] Karaloğlu F, Kemaloğlu YK, Yilmaz M, Ulukavak Çiftçi T, Çiftçi B, Bakkal FK. Comparison of full-night and ambulatory polysomnography with ApneaGraph in the subjects with obstructive sleep apnea syndrome. Eur Arch Otorhinolaryngol. 2017; 274(1):189–195

[13] Wall AJ, Arkwright JK, Reynolds K, et al. A multimodal optical catheter for diagnosing obstructive sleep apnea. Paper presented at: Optical Fibers and Sensors for Medical Diagnostics and Treatment Applications XIX2019; San Francisco

Index

Note: Page numbers set **bold** or *italic* indicate headings or figures, respectively.

Index